*O*vercoming Impotence

"This is the most comprehensive, practical book of its kind that I have seen written on erectile dysfunction. This book is an invaluable resource for interested laypersons coping with this medical condition."

—L. Dean Knoll, M.D.
Medical Director
Center for Urological Treatment and Research
Nashville, Tennessee

"Never before has such comprehensive and state-of-the-art medical information been so inviting and enjoyable. This superbly written guide appeals to all, from the afflicted to the curious. It has become an integral part of my treatment algorithm."

—Christopher S. Ng, M.D.
Endourology and Laparoscopic Urology
Cedars-Sinai Endourology Institute
Los Angeles, California

"[Dr. Jones] does an extraordinary job of presenting information about a difficult subject in a very readable and comfortable manner, . . . introducing humor and interesting anecdotal stories without detracting from the serious mission of the book—to inform men about a commonly misunderstood and underappreciated problem."

—Joseph A. Smith Jr., M.D.
Professor and Chairman
Department of Urologic Surgery
Vanderbilt University Medical Center
Nashville, Tennessee

"*Overcoming Impotence*, by J. Stephen Jones, is a very readable book with the subject presented in a complete and compassionate manner. . . . Dr. Jones speaks to what is normal and thereby dispels many myths about the subject. He also addresses medical and surgical methods of therapy, indicating their strengths and weaknesses. The book is thorough, and I believe it will serve as an excellent resource for anyone who is interested in learning about sexual dysfunction."

—W. Scott McDougal, M.D.
Walter S. Kerr Jr. Professor of Urology
Harvard Medical School
Chief of Urology
Massachusetts General Hospital

Overcoming Impotence

A Leading Urologist
Tells You Everything
You Need to Know

J. STEPHEN JONES, M.D.

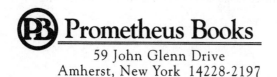 **Prometheus Books**

59 John Glenn Drive
Amherst, New York 14228-2197

Published 2003 by Prometheus Books

Inquiries should be addressed to
Prometheus Books
59 John Glenn Drive
Amherst, New York 14228–2197
VOICE: 716–691–0133, ext. 207
FAX: 716–564–2711
WWW.PROMETHEUSBOOKS.COM

07 06 05 04 03   5 4 3 2 1

Library of Congress Cataloging-in-Publication Data

Jones, J. Stephen, 1937–
     Overcoming impotence : a leading urologist tells you everything you need
to know / J. Stephen Jones.
          p. cm.
     Includes bibliographical references.
     ISBN 1–59102–128–6 (alk. paper)
     1. Impotence. 2. Consumer education. I. Title.

RC889.J56 2003
616.6'922—dc22

                                                                              2003018604

Printed in the United States of America on acid-free paper

To my family:

To Jared, who finally discovered the *power of the pen*.
You are the best of me and so much more. Reach for the stars.

To Katie, the real writer of the family—may the words continue
to spring from your spirit in order to enlighten ours.

And to Kathryn—words could not express the gratitude and esteem.

Contents

PART ONE: UNDERSTANDING IMPOTENCE: THIS NEVER HAPPENED TO ME BEFORE

CHAPTER 1: YOU'RE NOT THE FIRST TO PASS THIS WAY: IMPOTENCE THROUGHOUT HISTORY   31

CHAPTER 2: INTRODUCTION TO THE PENIS: THE LONG AND SHORT OF IT   37

CHAPTER 3: SECONDARY SEX ORGANS: BOYZ UNDER THE HOOD   49

CHAPTER 4: THE NORMAL ERECTION: WHAT COULD GO WRONG?   69

CHAPTER 5: WHO ARE THOSE PEOPLE ON TELEVISION? NORMAL SEXUAL FUNCTION   79

CHAPTER 6: WHY ME, LORD? CAUSES OF ERECTILE DYSFUNCTION 99

CHAPTER 7: DIAGNOSING IMPOTENCE: IT'S NOT HARD 127

CHAPTER 8: IT TAKES TWO TO TANGO: FEMALE SEXUALITY 147

CHAPTER 12: WHEN AN APPLE A DAY ISN'T ENOUGH: MEDICAL THERAPY 219

CHAPTER 13: PENILE INJECTION THERAPY: RISE AND SHINE   235

CHAPTER 14: RAISING THE BAR: PENILE PROSTHESES   249

Acknowledgments

The function of the teacher is to teach and to propagate the best that is known and taught in the world. To teach the current knowledge of the subject he professes.
—William Osler, *Teacher and Student*, 1892

*T*his book would have never reached fruition without the support and advice of several people critical to the process.

Although he will be described in the history books as one of the great statesmen of our era, the courage Senator Bob Dole demonstrated in sharing his own experiences—and successes—with the public will make perhaps an equally lasting impact. As the first man of such stature to openly discuss erectile dysfunction as a medical condition, Senator Dole eliminated a taboo. This milestone was critical to our journey toward successfully overcoming erectile dysfunction.

Linda Greenspan Regan at Prometheus Books seized on to the concept early on, and her enthusiasm became infectious. Her faith in my writing brought out the best.

Through the vision and support of Dr. Andrew C. Novick, the environment of the Glickman Urological Institute of the Cleveland Clinic Foundation allows talented people to reach their potential: I am a direct beneficiary of this environment. I appreciate the friendship and professionalism of all my staff and colleagues, with special thanks to Dr. Drogo K. Montague, who has kindly written the preface to this book. He was one of the pioneers that took the science of erectile dysfunction from its dark ages, when impotence was presumed to be "in the head," to its current status, where no man has to endure erectile dysfunction if motivated to overcome it. Men worldwide owe a debt to those pioneers, embodied at the Institute by Dr. Montague.

Nancy Mart, Shelly Kovacevic, and Jackie Johnson made sure I remained productive. Sandy Ausmundson is the ultimate professional as our impotence coordinator. The wonderful women at the Shaker Heights Public Library were always helpful, and professionally dealt with the titles of all the books I checked out to research this topic with few blushes.

My mother, Mary Jones, taught me from an early age to treasure the written word. The only thing she ever encouraged me more to pursue was the practice of medicine. With this book, her two aspirations for me have collided. I trust she sees her influence herein. My grandmother, Betty Young, is the matriarch every family should have—undoubtedly the kindest person ever to live. My father, Gene Jones, told me from childhood that my writing experiences would pay off someday, no matter what direction my career took. I hope he feels that day has arrived.

Finally, I thank Kathy, Jared, and Katie, to whom the book is dedicated.

FOREWORD

Senator Bob Dole
Former Senate majority leader
and 1996 presidential nominee

"*D*on't do it. You will be ridiculed, the butt of bad jokes—and you will be sorry!"

This was the advice I received when thinking about doing a commercial—not endorsing a product, but encouraging men to see a doctor if they were dealing with erectile dysfunction, commonly known as impotence.

Well, I did a commercial, and ridicule and jokes on late-night TV followed, but I also received countless thank-yous from men and women.

The bottom line is that we now speak publicly about something that was considered taboo just a few years ago. The benefits of this change in attitude are obvious, and the benefactors, both men and women, are grateful.

This book, *Overcoming Impotence*, by Dr. J. Stephen Jones of the Cleveland Clinic Foundation Urological Institute, gives you the full story, from causes to cures. It may be more than you ever want to know, but it is written in a way that makes it quite easy to understand. The book is not just about treatment but also about prevention of ED, or impotence.

My comments are those of a volunteer who has come to understand the problem and wants others to benefit from all the information Dr. Jones provides.

So, my advice: read this book and see your doctor!

Preface

Drogo K. Montague, M.D.
Director, Center for Sexual Function
Glickman Urological Institute
Cleveland Clinic Foundation

I received my medical degree in 1968. Knowledge concerning male sexual dysfunction at that time was sparse and is summarized from the following entry in the urology text I had used as a medical student, the fifth edition of D. R. Smith's *General Urology*:

> Various degrees of impotence in men are common, but it is rare to find definite organic cause for the complaints, which include inability to gain an erection, weak erections, premature ejaculation, loss of libido, or loss of normal sensation with ejaculation. The cause of almost all of these difficulties is psychogenic. . . .
>
> With few exceptions, the causes of sexual difficulties in the male are psychic, i.e., based on guilt, anxiety, jealousy, or frigidity on the part of the wife. . . . Many of these men are obviously tense and nervous. . . . Unless the patient's difficulties are of short duration, he should be referred to a psychiatrist.[1]

Interest on the part of urologists or any other members of the medical profession in either understanding the causes of male sexual dysfunction or in treating them remained almost nonexistent until effective treatment became available. Three major events have marked the history of male sexual dysfunction. They include the invention of the inflatable penile prosthesis in 1973, the concept of injecting erection-promoting drugs into the penis in 1983, and the marketing of Viagra in 1998.

D. R. Smith's text is still in use and is now in its fifteenth edition. In contrast to the two meager paragraphs that were present in the 1966 fifth edition, this current general urology text devotes an entire 23-page chapter as an introduction to this subject. Indeed, the body of knowledge concerning male sexual dysfunction has advanced to the state where entire textbooks have been written. These texts are an excellent source of information for the medical health professional but are not the best source of information for lay people. Although there are other books on this subject for the public, few are as comprehensive or as authoritative as this one authored by my friend and colleague, Steve Jones, and none are presented in as entertaining manner. Knowledge is power: enjoy your reading!

Dr. Montague is also a past president of the Sexual Medicine Society of North America and currently serves as chairman of the American Urological Association (AUA) Erectile Dysfunction Guidelines Committee.

Introduction

Thirty Million Men and Growing

The Club You Didn't Ask to Join

If sex is such a natural phenomenon, how come there are so many books on how to do it?

—Bette Midler

*F*orget all the jokes—sexual health is important. It plays a role in physical and mental well being that is as vital as almost any other bodily function. Sexual health is critical to reproduction. On an everyday basis, it has a profound impact on most adults' quality of life. Without sexual health, the species would be wiped out—*and life would be nowhere near as enjoyable.*

Unfortunately, society and medicine have openly acknowledged this fact only within the past few years. Doctors consequently had little to offer men suffering with erectile dysfunction throughout most of a long and unsatisfying history. Erections were poorly understood, so effective treatments were not available. Therefore, the conclusion was usually drawn that erectile dysfunction must be due to mental, not physical causes. All too often, men were told it was their fault (or their wives' fault) if they couldn't achieve an erection.

We now know that is simply not true.

There has never been a better time to have erectile dysfunction. Not that this fate should be wished on anyone, but at least *we can now successfully treat virtually all cases.* Whereas men with erectile dysfunction were disregarded in years past, because medicine was unable to help them, we can now offer multiple effective treatment options. Men who don't respond to oral medications can be treated through several other medical and surgical approaches that are covered in detail in this book. Indeed, it is a rare man that can't resume sexual activity if he and his partner are motivated. Yes, you were motivated enough to pick up this book, so read on to find the keys to a long, happy, and, most importantly, healthy sex life.

DEFINING ERECTILE DYSFUNCTION

Although chapter 7 explores in depth the various scientific definitions of erectile dysfunction, for now, let's keep it simple: *It doesn't work.* In other words, if a man or his partner is dissatisfied with the quality, endurance, or anything else about his erection, he can be said to have *erectile dysfunction.*

We used to break down erectile dysfunction into two groups—*psychogenic* or *physical.* We now know, however, that almost all cases involve at least some component of each. Importantly, whereas we formerly believed a majority of cases to be psychologically based, we now know the opposite is true. Most men who experience difficulties with erections have underlying physical problems. Overcoming these physical limitations can yield results that can permanently restore sexual satisfaction.

Finally, many of you will wonder what the difference is between *erectile dysfunction* and *impotence.* There is none. The term erectile dysfunction arose in the early nineties to counteract the negative connotation of the term *impotence.* Impotence literally means "without power," so some people felt it presented patients in a negative light. *Erectile dysfunction* became popularized when it entered the lay lexicon in association with the marketing campaign for Viagra. You will note that I use the terms somewhat interchangeably throughout this book. Although the politically correct term *erectile dysfunction* is the preferred term, the less cumbersome *impotence* is more commonly understood. Its familiarity to the public and conciseness are the reasons it was chosen for the title of this book. For the same reasons it will be used in many circumstances that we will explore.

INTERNATIONAL DIFFERENCES

Sex in America is an obsession. In other parts of the world a fact.
—Marlene Dietrich

According to Ridwan Shabsigh, M.D., a presenter at a recent gathering of the American Urological Association (AUA), men from different cultures deal with erectile dysfunction very differently. American men, products of the most medicalized society on earth, are motivated to find a cure. They more often want to know that there is an anatomical reason for their problems. Americans are more likely to want the problem corrected, not just treated one night at a time. They expect something like the computer programs that are now available that will take the hard drive back to a time before the crash. However, no such software exists for this hardware. Despite their willingness to look for physical causes, American men are less likely than others to consider their erectile dysfunction to have a psychological component. Therefore, they are less likely to deal with the psychological issues that inevitably play some role.

As lovers of legendary status, French men are supposed to be the most embarrassed by erectile dysfunction. However, they are less likely than Americans to pursue medical intervention or surgery. Their approach is often a belief that the natural state of the body is to be maintained. Considering the fact that smoking is the number one cause of erectile dysfunction, their societal chain-smoking is counterintuitive to keeping the body in its natural state.

German men are apparently most prepared to deal rationally with their condition, exhibiting the least depression or angst. On the contrary, Italians are completely unwilling to accept erectile dysfunction. The burden of the image of the "Italian Stallion" leaves little room for tolerating sexual problems. Finally, Spanish men rationalize that their diminishing erections are simply due to a loss of interest in sex. If they can't have it, they reason, they don't want it.

AM I ALONE?

Is it not strange that desire should so many years outlive performance?
—Shakespeare, *Henry IV*, act 2, scene 4

A common sentiment experienced by any man when he first encounters difficulties with erections is the feeling that he's the only man he knows to have ever experienced such a problem. Due to societal prejudices about the importance of sexual potency, most men who notice weakening erections don't rush to tell their friends about it. Likewise, the friends don't tell anyone either. That can lead to the erroneous conclusion that you're the only guy that you know who has erectile dysfunction. Not even close!

Up to thirty million American men are affected at the present time.[1] More new cases arise (or don't arise!) every day, on the order of 600,000–700,000 new cases each year. That means that almost two thousand American men roll over every night and say, "This never happened to me before." Even so, most of these men have not yet sought treatment.

The incidence goes up substantially with age, increasing significantly above the age of sixty-five—which is rapidly approaching for the baby boomers. Although erectile dysfunction becomes more likely with advancing age, there is certainly no age cutoff for a sexually fulfilling life. Some men enjoy sexual activity into their eighties and nineties.

Although impossible to document, almost every adult male experiences at least one occasion when he is not satisfied with the outcome. When surveyed, at least 50 percent will complain of difficulties at some point in life about some degree of erectile insufficiency. The definitive research quoted is the *Massachusetts Male Aging Study*, published in 1994.[2] This survey was the first comprehensive look at sexual activity since the Kinsey survey forty years earlier.[3] The researchers studied 1,290 men and found that over half of them complained of some degree of erectile dysfunction. This was broken down into those with minimal (17 percent), moderate (25 percent) or severe (10 percent) erectile dysfunction.

Strikingly, almost 40 percent of the men had some degree of erectile dysfunction by the age of *forty*. By the time their subjects reached seventy, two-thirds of them reported erectile dysfunction. These percentages represent huge numbers of men of a similar age in society.

Moreover, if you add in cofactors like heart disease, diabetes, high blood pressure, ulcers, arthritis, and allergies, the percentage of men with erectile dysfunction went up even higher. The same thing was found among men taking medications in several categories. Psychological factors that increased risk or erectile dysfunction included depression, excessive alcohol use, and anger.

The greatest risk factor of all was found to be smoking. Smokers were almost three times as likely as nonsmokers to be completely unable to achieve an erection. (The role of all these risk factors and causes is explored in chapter 6.)

Thus, the incidence of erectile dysfunction is huge, perhaps as high as 150 million men worldwide. Assuming two-thirds of men have at least some trouble by the age of seventy as shown in the *Massachusetts Male Aging Study*, most men will experience problems if they live long enough. That doesn't have to be discouraging news, however. Instead, it should let you know that you're not alone. Be sure to speak up to your physician if there is a problem. Help is readily available, so you are only alone if *you* choose to be.

WHAT CAN THIS BOOK DO FOR ME?

This book is designed to help you overcome erectile dysfunction. For men who aren't currently having difficulties, that may mean prevention. For men having mild erectile dysfunction, it may mean heading things off at the pass. Finally, for men who can't achieve or maintain an adequate erection, it may mean receiving treatment. There is help available for all three groups of men.

Physicians aren't always the best communicators. In order to overcome that tendency, I have made every effort to make this book accessible to all readers. Although we must use many words that may initially be unfamiliar to you, each of them will be demystified. Each term in **bold** from this point on is defined in the text and then redefined in the Definition of Terms section, following the conclusion. In order to avoid repeatedly redefining these medical terms, the reader may want to check that section to reinforce his memory. In addition, at many points in the book the reader will be referred to another chapter in order to avoid repetition.

The first few chapters are targeted to help you understand erectile dysfunction by introducing the normal anatomy and function of the male sex organs. Next comes an explanation of the numerous things that can go wrong and the ways we can evaluate these problems. The end of the first section explores the female role in erectile dysfunction, as well as female sexuality; it concludes with a discussion of what you might expect from a visit to the urologist.

The second section is dedicated to treatment, ranging from simple to complex: from nonprescription remedies to complex surgery; from aphrodisiacs to Zoloft. With so many treatments available to successfully overcome erectile dysfunction, there is no reason for you to suffer silently with this problem.

Finally, please bear in mind that the men and women discussed in this book are real people, patients who have shared intimate details of their lives. Although their names and identifying details have been changed, their stories are genuine. My understanding of sexual function and dysfunction is richer because they and thousands of others have opened up to their physician. I hope their experiences help enrich your life similarly.

Part One

Understanding Impotence

This Never Happened to Me Before

You're Not the First to Pass This Way

Impotence throughout History

When a man tells you he's too old to get it up, you better watch out, son. He's probably sleeping with your wife.
—Smead Wright, Ozarkian sage

IN THE BEGINNING . . .

*R*eferences to **impotence** can be found truly from the beginning. Genesis has the original description of the malady that God used for preventing not-so-original sin.[1] In this passage, King Abimelech tried to seduce Abraham's wife, Sarah. God could have struck him down when caught in the transgression, but instead, struck down only his erections. He became the first man we know of who found himself not up to the occasion when God "*suffered thee not to touch her.*" (The Lord giveth, and the Lord taketh away.) The distressed king probably told Sarah the standard line, "This never happened to me before." Of course, it had never happened to *anyone* before.

Far more forgiving than most men, Abraham asked God to restore the King's potency. The Maker obliged and became the real Father of urology,* imparting a cure for impotence long before Bob Dole introduced us to his "little blue friend." Abraham and Sarah moved on, just to be safe.

---

*No disrespect intended to Dr. Hugh Hampton Young, the father of modern urology.

Impotence reappeared soon thereafter, when God caught King David cheating with Bathsheba. Hoping to hide his impregnation of Bathsheba, David summoned her husband, Uriah, home from war for a conjugal visit. The plan was to convince the Hittite warrior that Bathsheba's child was conceived while Uriah was on weekend pass. Observing the legend of boxers and soldiers—that sex before competition weakens the warrior— Uriah resisted the offer. When David saw his plan failing, he got Uriah inebriated and sent him home. The drunken warrior maintained nerves of steel and slept on the front porch to avoid temptation.

No longer able to hide paternity, King David sent Uriah to certain death on the battlefield. Remembering God's punishment for Abimelech, David soon found himself in the same predicament. Without Abraham there to pray for David, this King resorted to an impotence treatment more common at the time. His servants brought him a "very fair . . . young virgin . . . that my lord may get heat." The ingénue, Abishag, "ministered to him, but the king knew her not." Unable to raise his sword in the bedroom, he was judged unfit to lead and was relieved of his crown as well.[2]

AFTER GENESIS

> Suddenly, instead of the fire that devoured me, I felt a deathly cold flow through my veins; my legs trembled; I sat down on the point of fainting and wept like a child.
> —Jean-Jacques Rousseau, describing his first impotence episode

Early descriptions of erectile dysfunction can be found on Egyptian papyrus dating to around 2000 B.C.E. These writings describe two types of impotence: the first was "natural impotence," meaning the man was simply incapable of an erection. The second, more difficult, type was "supernatural," the result of evil influence or sorcery.

Impotence in the seventeenth century changed the face of Western civilization. The Spanish Hapsburg Empire reigned supreme over much of the world for centuries. Their downfall was attributed to the impotence of their final leader. Unable to keep it up long enough to propagate the lineage, Don Carlos II sought all available impotence treatments including exorcisms (seventeenth-century psychotherapy). Since his impotence endured, the Hapsburg lineage—and empire—did not.

Other historical figures rumored impotent include Kings Richard I and

Louis XVI, George Bernard Shaw, Sigmund Freud, Napoleon, Beethoven, and Rousseau. Rousseau's 1762 essay "Discourse on the Arts and Sciences" argued that the advancement of science and medicine had not been beneficial to mankind. He would have felt differently had the FDA approved Viagra in the eighteenth century. Edgar Allen Poe's most famous line, "Nevermore," evidently referred to his love life.

Curiously absent from the list of rumored impotent men from history are American presidents. Apparently, no one has trouble with erections while living in the White House—at least not the lack of them.

HISTORY: CAUSES

The psychological basis for impotence was recognized in Greek mythology when Iphiclus, son of King Phylacus, couldn't fulfill his princely duties. A mythological urologist, Melampus, took on the case. He discovered that a young Iphiclus had witnessed his own father, bloody knife in hand, turning one of the royal steeds into a royal gelding. After confronting his fear of castration, the prince recovered fully. The gelding did not.

Hippocrates believed two things caused most erectile dysfunction: a preoccupation with business combined with a lack of attraction to the man's female partner. Through the 1970s the prevailing opinion in urology texts was that "impotence, although mostly psychogenic," was still largely related to the stress of overworking. "Life is a competitive struggle," stated the most significant urological textbook of the time. "It may be ambition which is making them work too hard."[3] The rat race that Hippocrates first described persists. Early urological texts usually chose discretion in refusing comment on the female attractiveness part. In addition, he believed the rich were more likely to be impotent due to horseback riding. This may have been more accurate than we previously believed, based on recent findings of increased impotence among bicycle riders.

Although we now know that most cases of impotence have physical causes, modern medicine practically ignored this possibility until the 1980s. Of almost three thousand pages in the 1970 edition of *Campbell's Urology* (the bible of urology), less than four were devoted to impotence. Twice as many were dedicated to masturbation. It is a testament to the advancement of urology, and probably as importantly to the aging baby boomer population, that the most recent edition devotes well over one hundred pages to impotence. Omitting most of the section on masturbation freed up some space.

HISTORY: TREATMENT

Before urologists recognized the physical nature of impotence, treatments generally fell into three categories—aphrodisiacs, surgery/transplants, and mechanical treatments.

Aphrodisiacs

Innumerable substances have been used to increase sexual performance. Oysters, lobsters, eggs, and spices are examples. Spanish Fly, a substance made by grinding the wings of certain beetles, was a favorite of that party animal, the Marquis de Sade. It is illegal in the United States both because of the unproven nature of its effectiveness and a tendency to cause seizures or death. Many of these substances actually do nothing more than irritate the genital organs. The user interprets this irritation as increased sensitivity, thereby giving the impression of increased performance.

Rhinoceros horn has been used (unsuccessfully) for so long that its name has become synonymous with sexual arousal. Unfortunately, its popularity has led to such widespread slaughter of the animals that they face extinction.

Ancient Egyptians believed eating crocodile penises increased virility. Anyone capable of eating a crocodile's penis probably didn't need any more help proving his manhood.

Surgery/Transplants

The idea of using animal testes to treat impotence began in the Middle Ages, when a standard treatment for "the male malady" was to place the testicles of a cock under the bed. Another option was eating the rooster's testes. You could guess that putting them under the bed was much more popular. The *Malleus Maleficarum* was a guide to witchcraft during that era that asserted witch's spells caused impotence. This was a major reason witch-hunting became so widespread.

French physiologist Charles Edouard Brown-Sequard injected himself in the 1880s with an extract from the testicles of dogs that he claimed made him smarter, stronger, and more virile. After ten injections, he reported improved erections, as well as a stronger jet of urine and "power of defe-cation." He made no claims about the effect this had on the dogs. His "Elixir of Life" became an instant best-seller. Its 1889 launch rivaled that of Viagra, even without a famous spokesman.

Eugen Steinach in 1920 pioneered surgical treatment of impotence with a revolutionary idea—**vasectomy**. He believed blocking the **vas deferens** (the tubes **semen** passes through) would force maleness factors back into the bloodstream instead of letting them go to waste on the sheets. The erections probably weren't much better, but with female partners spending less time pregnant, there was much more opportunity. Two recipients of the Steinach procedure were Sigmund Freud and Nobel Prize winner William Butler Yeats. Freud, the person most responsible for the mistaken impression that impotence was primarily psychological, set back our understanding of the disorder by decades. Taking him out of the gene pool probably did more to help the science of impotence therapy than anything else Steinach did.

Many respected universities have subsequently been involved in the transplantation of animal or human testicular tissue. Swiss professor Paul Niehans treated tens of thousands of men with testicular cell injections in the early twentieth century. His procedure sometimes went straight to the root of the problem by injecting a booster shot directly into the patient's testes.* Patients receiving the treatments included Charlie Chaplin (and you wondered why he walked that way), Aristotle Onassis, and Pope Pius XII. Chaplin was a well-known womanizer, but the Pope's interest in this treatment remains a mystery. Another researcher in Chicago proudly stated his initial patient checked himself out of the hospital four days after surgery in order to satisfy his newfound potency. He fully understood the rule: "Never waste an erection."

Dr. Leo Stanley removed the testicles of recently executed prisoners at San Quentin in the 1920s. He transplanted them into other, more fortunate (albeit impotent) prisoners, reporting improvement in strength, well-being, and libido among the recipients. When the supply ran low, he substituted goat, ram, boar, and deer testicular tissue. Why he wanted to improve libido among prisoners is still not evident.

It remains unclear whether any of these early attempts at treating impotence with human or animal testicular tissue actually worked. Most of the researchers mentioned eventually fell into disrepute—but at least Aristotle Onassis got the girl.

---

*Ouch.

Mechanical

Hot metal rods inserted into the **urethra** during medieval times failed to revive erections. No one wanted a second treatment, so failures went unreported. Many types of splints have been used, including hollowed-out antlers and horns.

Encouraged by finding the penis bone (baculum) in some animals, early surgeons placed rib cartilage into the penis. Although these initial attempts failed, penile prostheses (see chapter 14) have more recently proven particularly reliable.

KEY POINTS

- Erectile dysfunction has been around as long as mankind has been dysfunctional.
- Treatment has only become feasible in the past few decades.
- The "good old days" weren't so good for men with erectile dysfunction.

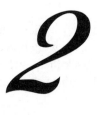

Introduction to the Penis

The Long and Short of It

God gave us all a penis and a brain, but only enough blood to run one at a time.

—Robin Williams

*S*ome people don't consider the penis a vital organ. Those are the people that don't have one. The rest find the penis an enigmatic body part—a source of potentially endless wonderment and entertainment. However, if its vitality were truly endless, we wouldn't need this book, would we?

THE NORMAL PENIS: SIZE MATTERS

"Phallacies" abound regarding the penis. Size is the usually the biggest focus. Despite widely held assumptions about differences in penis size, remarkably little is actually known about what normal size is. Innumerable jokes abound on penis size, as does daily banter between men of every geographic and socioeconomic group. Usually unspoken, penis size is seen as a surrogate for importance or power.

It matters.

However, the medical literature has remarkably little documentation of normal penile length. Urology textbooks don't even acknowledge that anyone would care to know. The earliest known report on penis size was in

1879, when Krause concluded average erect length was $8\frac{1}{4}$ inches. The scant research available more recently indicates Krause's eyes were bigger than his topic really was. Or maybe penises were bigger back then—when men were men. More recent studies show the average length of the erect male penis to be almost five inches.

Brazilian urologists in the nineties presented a study on the topic at the American Urological Association (AUA) Annual Meeting. These adventurous physicians determined average erect length to be 5.7 inches (ranging from 3.5–7.5 inches) in Brazil. I joined hundreds of other inquiring urological minds attending this presentation to witness the unveiling of cutting-edge data. We expected their findings to finally answer the big question. However, we neglected to take into account that most urologists are males. Instead of a spirited intellectual debate, the only meaty discussion involved a group of French urologists demanding that, had the study been performed in France, the measurements would have been much larger. Boys—even grown urologists gathered for the world's largest gathering of urological minds—will be boys. The Great French-Brazilian Penis War was the highlight of that year's convention.

The Kinsey study on sexual behavior was one of three that asked men to measure and report their own penis size. Their most significant finding was that men lie about the size of their penises.

Really.

We have even less information about girth. The World Health Organization did its own study because of complaints by British men that government-approved condoms were too tight. The British standard requires the condom to measure 52 mm (about 2 inches) wide when placed flat on a table. They found over one-third of the penises in Britain didn't fit. Maybe that will quiet the French once and for all.

The sixteenth-century Indian book of love, the *Kama Sutra*, describes three kinds of men based on penis size. Hares are defined as having penile length of six fingers. Bulls are eight fingers long, Stallions twelve. We must assume the fingers are side-by-side, not lengthways.

DOES SIZE *REALLY* MATTER?

> Of the virile member when it is hard, it is thick and long, dense and heavy, and when it is limp, it is thin, short of flesh or wind but to arterial blood.
>
> —Leonardo da Vinci

Traditional thinking has been that size really doesn't matter. ("It's not the size of the wand; it's the magic with which you wave it.") Although many suspect this is the kind of logic men with small penises have, it really is true regarding the sexual enjoyment of both the male and his partner. The vaginal diameter can stretch from zero (most of the time the walls are collapsed together) to huge (about the time junior's head passes through). With this adaptability, it makes sense that female partners report no difference in either pleasure or discomfort in men they judge to have larger or smaller penises.

Women perceive essentially no sexual stimulation anywhere in the **vagina** except in the third that is closest to the exterior. Assuming even the smallest penis will reach one-third of the way in, no man should feel unfit. In fact, most women get more stimulation in the clitoris, which is outside the vagina entirely. Any man incapable of reaching the **clitoris** is simply not trying.

It is widely assumed that race or ethnicity defines penis size. The second half of this assumption that many people have is that white men have smaller flaccid penises that simply enlarge more during erection, evening the playing field when it really counts. Because of the controversial—and trivial—nature of the question, we'll probably never get a good scientific study on racial differences in penis size. The only research reporting any indication that black men have larger penises is the British Flat Condom Study. Only 14 percent of white men found the condoms too small, whereas 38 percent of black men did. Indirect evidence, but about all there is beyond locker-room humor.

IT PAYS TO BE BORN IN THE RIGHT ERA

> The organ has been venerated, reviled, and misrepresented with intent in art, literature, and legend through the centuries.
> —William H. Masters and Virginia E. Johnson,
> *Human Sexual Response*, 1960

The Athenians of ancient Greece actually valued the smaller, "dainty" penis. Their culture was recorded primarily through artwork, where the penis was depicted large only on characters that would be considered vulgar or evil. The politicians in charge apparently all had tiny penises. This prerequisite may persist.

Unfortunately, the media have unduly influenced our perception of penis size. Insecurities are exposed by doctored images of porn stars like

Johnny Holmes. Long Dong Silver's penis was Exhibit 1 at the Clarence Thomas Senate confirmation hearings. It's not accidental these men with seemingly impressive organs are the ones shown in the movies. What other line of work does "well-hung" qualify one for? These men are always shown from creative photographic angles—never coming from a cold shower.

The bottom line is that the penis should be large enough to do its job. It should be long enough to deposit **semen** into the vaginal vault. It should be long enough to miss the toilet lid. Anything else is window dressing.

PENILE ENLARGEMENT: MAKING THE WORST OF A BAD SITUATION

> The functioning role of the penis is as well established as that of any other organ in the body. Ironically, there is no organ about which more misinformation has been perpetrated.
> —Masters and Johnson, *Human Sexual Response*

Mitch is a 32-year-old stocky salesman, unsure of himself on several fronts. He requested information on penile enlargement surgery because he thought his penis was too short. Recently divorced, he had joined a health club and was self-conscious both in the showers at the club and with his new girlfriend.

On examination, his stretched penis length was 4.5 inches from the pubic bone to the tip, just less than average length. He also admitted about 30 pounds weight gain since graduating high school.

When informed that his penis length was about average, and would appear to be even longer if it didn't have the beer belly hiding it, he was not completely reassured. Fortunately, the cost of penile enlargement surgery took away his enthusiasm for the procedure. With the 20-pound weight loss he achieved over the next few months, his body image improved dramatically, and he lost all interest in the operation.

Insecure males came out of the woodwork in the nineties with the emergence of penile enlargement surgery. Comedian Flip Wilson championed the wonders of the procedure on the Howard Stern Show in 1997. Mercifully, he didn't show as much on the program as Howard sometimes convinces his guests to do. A longer penis clearly doesn't lead to a longer life. Mr. Wilson died the following year.

Although the idea of easily gaining a few inches obviously appeals to some men, most urologists have not been impressed with these procedures. Complications abound, including severe or potentially life-threatening infections. We urologists who don't perform these procedures only see the patients when things turn bad and after they have left their doctors, of course. By then, they are often miserable and embarrassed to the point they may deny they've had surgery, even when confronted with the evidence of sutures all over the penis.

Their embarrassment is justified. First, this is an experimental procedure that has not been adequately researched. Second, most of these patients only *believe* that their penis is too small to trigger the automatic flusher in a public restroom. They usually have psychologically—not physically—small penises. Surgery doesn't cure psychological inadequacy.

Success with these procedures is deemed great if the penile length is increased by even an inch. And of course the penologists doing the surgery wouldn't fudge their before-and-after measurements, would they? Don't be surprised if we begin to see a semi-pornographic version of those before and after diet ads. To add insult to injury, many doctors performing these procedures prescribe the use of penile weights to stretch the newly renovated unit. These are supposed to add a little extra length each time they do penis weightlifting—or weightholding.

Advocates claim the greatest benefit is in the flaccid, not erect length, enabling these men to feel better while changing in the locker room. Anyone bothered by other guys looking at his penis in the locker room should probably find a new health club.

IN SEARCH OF THE HIDDEN PENIS

In addition to those with insecurities, obese men are the other target group for penile lengthening surgery. These men don't really have a short penis. They just have a suprapubic fat pad (the second belly many develop covering the pubic bone) hiding most of the penis. At least these men have some improvement in apparent length, even if it's just smoke and mirrors. This is because the penis is like a tree; about half is "underground" normally, extending into the body and anchoring on the pelvic bones. This part is literally called the *root*, proving anatomists have a sense of humor after all. Exposing a few inches of hidden penis by removing the fat around it obviously makes the tree trunk appear more substantial.

The first thing for these men to consider is that their penis is normal-sized; it's just that more than half of it is buried inside their oversized bodies. This knowledge should validate these men's manhood and make them more interested in weight loss than penile enlargement surgery, but as you may guess, it usually doesn't.

Some of the suprapubic fat that is surgically removed from around the tree trunk is sometimes wrapped around the penis (under the bark, if you will), in order to increase the girth. This actually creates the most unappealing aspect of the operation as the body unevenly reabsorbs the dead fat. This creates the lumpy-bumpy appearance of a bratwurst after heating on the grill. (Drives the girls wild.) Another site for donor fat to thicken the penis is the buttock. Nothing I could add would make that mental image any better.

Additional length is gained by cutting the penile *suspensory ligament.* Back to the tree analogy, this structure is like the guy-wire that keeps a newly planted tree from falling over in the wind. Cutting the ligament is supposed to let the penis fall farther away from the body, giving it another millimeter or so of length. When this ligament is cut too much, the penis sometimes becomes unmanageable like those big balloons in a windy Thanksgiving Day parade. It gives new meaning to the phrase "Free Willy."

WHERE DID IT GO?

> The indocile liberty of this member [the penis] is very remarkable, so importunately unruly in its tumidity and impatience when we do not require it, and so unseasonably disobedient when we stand most in need of it.
>
> —Michel Eyquem de Montaigne, 1580

Most males who think their penis is shrinking, of course, have simply gained weight. This simply creates a situation where more of the penis is buried underground. However, shrinking of the penis is often suspected with aging. Although unproven, many urologists suspect there is some truth to the adage, "If you don't use it, you lose it." Or at least, if you don't use it, it shrinks. It appears that the increased blood flow of regular erections keeps the erectile tissue healthy and fully expanded. Some older men may develop shrinkage when erections become rare or absent. These men are usually beyond desire for sexual activity and aren't concerned by this minor change. Typically, they don't undress in locker rooms where men look at each other's penises either.

Koro is an anxiety condition, found usually along the Pacific Rim, where men believe their penis is shrinking. In Malay, the term means "head of a turtle," which visually describes the retraction these men fear is occurring. The Chinese term for koro is *suk yeong*. (No kidding.) This anxiety can be so overwhelming that the patient actually holds onto his penis to keep it from retracting into his body. Worse, some of these men may place wires, ropes, chopsticks or metal objects onto or through their penises to prevent retraction. Similar to the discussion above on penile enlargement surgery, these men have psychological, not physical issues.

Koro is a fascinating phenomenon that has caused widespread panic in several third world countries. A mass outbreak involving about 4,500 cases in Singapore in 1967–68 threatened social stability. Men with this condition in America usually just buy a sports car.

NORMAL PENILE ANATOMY: PARTS

> The glans is the extreme part of the Yard, soft and of an exquisite feeling . . . which moving up and down in the act of copulation, brings pleasure both to the man and woman.
> —Nicholas Culpepper, *A Directory for Midwives*, 1660

Males clearly fixate on their penises, but most don't really know what one consists of. Even physicians don't ordinarily study the organ in depth. Medical students spend a semester learning the brain, but only a few minutes in lecture cover the penis. *Gray's Anatomy* has more than twice as many pages on the nose as the penis. Illogical. When is the last time you heard men bragging about the size of their brain or nose?

The main bulk of the penis is composed of three tubes running lengthwise (see Fig. 1). On top are two side-by-side cylinders, each of which is called a **corpus cavernosum** (the plural of which is **corpora cavernosae**). During erection the corpora cavernosae fill with blood under pressure, kind of like inflating a tire, or maybe an inflatable raft. We often refer to the cavernosae as the **corporal bodies**. A tough coat called the **tunica albuginea** surrounds each corpus cavernosum, like the steel belt of the radial tire. Another layer called *Buck's fascia* wraps around both corpora cavernosae. (More proof anatomists have a sense of humor, contrary to popular wisdom.)

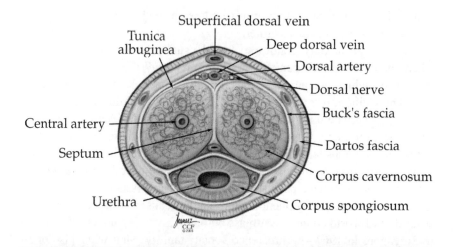

Fig. I. Penile anatomy.

Immediately below the corpora cavernosae runs the third tube, called the **corpus spongiosum**.* The **urethra** carries urine and semen through the spongiosum to the tip of the penis. Here, the *urethral meatus* (the anatomists' sense of humor at work again) forms a slit-like opening to the outside world. The spongiosum spreads out at the end of the penis to form the helmet-shaped **glans penis** or "head." The glans penis holds the nerve fibers that give the penis its sensitivity. The rounded rim of the glans penis is called the **corona**. (We must wonder what beer anatomists drink.)

A hood of skin (the *foreskin*) covers the glans penis at birth. Its medical name is the *prepuce*. This is such a bad name that urologists use it only when writing scientific papers, and try to not say it aloud because few are sure how to pronounce it. Circumcised men have had the prepuce removed. The *frenulum* is the web of skin on the underside that seems to connect the shaft to the glans penis. Modern science has found absolutely no use for this structure.

Despite the nickname for an erection, the human penis does not contain any bones. Some mammals have a bone called the *os penis* or *baculum*. The walrus baculum reaches over two feet long, which may have inspired John Lennon's line, "I am the walrus." In addition to making the male members of these species reliable in bed, these bones in ancient times were

---

*Fortunately, we don't have to learn the plural form of corpus spongiosum except in cases of a very rare duplication of the penis called *diphallus*. You don't want to know.

used for sewing needles or toothpicks. This explains why people in ancient times frequently let things remain stuck between their teeth.

Leonardo da Vinci believed humans had a similar bone: "The origin of the penis is situated upon the pubic bones so that it can resist its active force on coitus. If this bone did not exist the penis, in meeting resistance, would turn backward and would often enter more into the body of the operator than into the body of the operated."

The penis receives its blood supply from the **pudendal arteries** and veins. Once inside the penis, the arteries branch out and drain into **sinusoids**. These sacks can fill with pressure so the tire becomes inflated and rigid.

The *penile nerves* weren't fully understood until recently. These tiny strands of tissue are hard to see, so they're often overlooked by surgeons and anatomists alike. In 1981, Dr. Patrick Walsh was in the Netherlands to address a medical meeting. Since it was Dr. Walsh's birthday, his hosts reserved a free afternoon for any leisure activity he desired. Most people could think of dozens of things to do for a birthday party in the Netherlands; he chose to spend the afternoon in the anatomic dissection lab on the host university's campus exploring the exact route the nerves took through the pelvis en route to the penis. His discovery completely changed our understanding of this anatomy. Since we know where the nerves are located, we can now preserve them during urological surgery (see chapter 6). Already one of the preeminent urologists in the world, he thus secured his place in history.

And he didn't have a headache the next day.

A ROSE BY ANY OTHER NAME

For some reason many men refer to their penises in the third person. This often involves naming the organ, such as LBJ's comrade, "Jumbo." Most adolescent males name their penises at some point, reputedly because they don't want a stranger making decisions for them. Many don't outgrow it. Women never do anything like this, thankfully. A New York socialite apparently referred to her husband's as the Trump Tower. Willard reportedly snaked around the White House with Socks the cat.

Synonyms for the organ are said to outnumber almost any other word in the English language. Shakespeare is believed to have even slipped in his own euphemism when Rosalinde was "pricked" by a rose.* Discretion

---

*"He that sweetest rose will find / Must find love's prick and Rosalinde" (from *As You Like It*, act 3, scene 2).

limits discussion of the many variations on nicknames for the word. The only one too good to overlook is the term *dork*, which refers to a whale penis. The dork is rumored to approach ten feet long in some of the large sea mammals—true inspiration for Herman Melville's aptly named novel about a whale named Moby.

OTHER FAMOUS PENISES: WHERE ARE THEY NOW?

Few penises become famous enough to be discussed in Supreme Court nomination hearings. Nonetheless, some earn legendary status without the benefit of wide-angle lenses.

Egyptian mythology heralds the earliest missing-penis stories. Set (also known as Seth, believed to be the embodiment of the evil god Typhon) killed and dismembered his nephew Osiris. Literally. He scattered fourteen parts across Egypt, tossing the warrior's member into the Nile. Isis, Osiris's wife and sister, held the ultimate treasure hunt throughout the kingdom. She reassembled her husband when all but one of the parts was relocated. Unfortunately for Isis (and more unfortunately for Osiris), a crab had eaten Osiris's penis, so even when all the other body parts were reassembled and brought back to life, he was never again the man she married. Luckily, they already had a son from B.C. ("before castration") who exacted revenge by castrating the evil uncle. The crab's fate is unknown.

Legend has it that someone took Napoleon's "Bonaparte" before burial. A New York urologist reportedly paid $40,000 for the "parte." That seems like a lot considering the dictator was widely believed to be impotent, perhaps explaining why Josephine would let the parte out of the estate. A premonition of castration may have inspired him to keep his hand in that defensive position we all recognize.

Rasputin became known as "the great survivor" due to his many escapes from assassination attempts by those trying to get him out of the Russian royal household. He survived being poisoned, bludgeoned, run over, stabbed, and shot before meeting his end in the icy river Neva. Legend suggests the final insult was the removal of his well-traveled member, an act not even the great survivor could handle. A shriveled specimen made its rounds through the collectibles community, but its whereabouts now is unknown. (The media could do one of those "Where are they now?" specials.) The last known owner was a peasant woman in Paris who kept it in a velvet-lined wooden box.

A photo of outlaw John Dillinger's recently deceased body showed an impressive silhouette below the waist that carried his fame to new heights. It is still an area of disagreement as to whether the extraordinary outline was from his penis or simply his hands folded on his lap, but the former makes a much better story. Rumor had the FBI gathering this piece of evidence and placing it in the Smithsonian. The curators get multiple inquiries about this yearly but consistently deny possessing his six-shooter.

KEY POINTS

- There is no official word on penile size, but one of any size should do the job just fine.
- The penis is primarily composed of three cylinders: two for erection and one for urination. That could be interpreted to mean that it should spend twice as much time on sex as on urination.
- Several famous penises are missing and out of action.
- The properly functioning penis must do three things described in the following chapters: transmit sperm for reproduction, carry urine from the bladder to the outside world, and have an erection for recreational purposes with satisfactory frequency and reliability. If it doesn't do those things, read on.

3 Secondary Sex Organs
Boyz under the Hood

From the perspective of heterosexual production, the penis is just a
delivery system. But from the perspective of male pleasure, the penis
is everything: the alpha and omega, the beginning and the end.
—Gary Taylor

*I*f the penis is the center of a man's universe, then there are some
important planets nearby. Most other organs involved in male
sexual function are inside the scrotum—testicles and their cords—or the
pelvis—seminal vesicles and prostate. All these other players are known as
secondary sex organs. The secondary sex organs don't receive the attention
the penis gets when the topic is sex, but each plays its own key role.

TESTICLES: BOYZ WILL BE BOYZ

As vital organs go, the testicles are greatly under appreciated. These little
"balls" hanging behind the penis aren't impressive to look at, but carry
inside the future of the species. All mammalian life relies on some male
animal producing sperm to fertilize the female's eggs. This whole process
originates in the testicles (see Fig. 2).

The terms *testis* and *testicle* are interchangeable. *Etymologists*
(word historians) believe the words are based on the root meaning "to

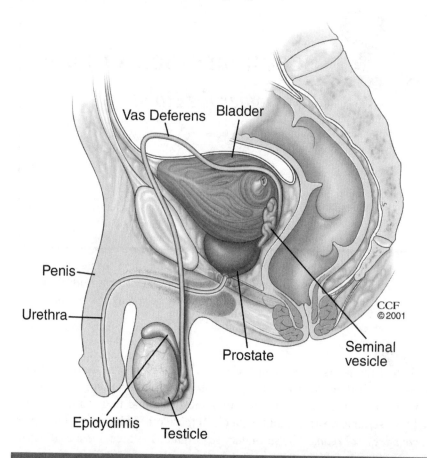

Fig. 2. Male pelvic anatomy.

testify." The Bible describes the tradition of putting one's hand on another man's testicles prior to testifying the truth. Abraham ordered his eldest house servant, "Put thy hand under my thigh, and I will make thee swear by the Lord, the God of heaven."[2] A case could be made that the Bible was transcribed into bound form so a witness would thereafter have a better place to put the hand for swearing the truth in court than someone else's testicles.

Unlike penises, testes aren't often the focus of size arguments. Most men have testicles 1½ to 2 inches long and about half that size in width and depth. The ram has the largest testicles on the planet in comparison to body weight. Interestingly, despite huge testes, the ram ejaculate is less than half the volume of humans, about one milliliter. The boar, despite smaller testes, ejaculates up to a liter.

The inside of each testis is packed tightly with tiny tubes that do nothing but crank out sperm all day. These tubes, called **seminiferous tubules**, are coils that can stretch out to about a yard long. One hundred of them could stretch the length of a football field, and all these tubules from one testis might stretch for miles if one took the time to line them all up.

Between the spaces in these coils are the **Leydig cells**—little cellular **testosterone** factories. Based on its control of these Leydig cells, the only male sexual organ under predictable control of the brain is the testis; testosterone production of these Leydig cells is turned on and off by the tiny *pituitary gland*. This tiny gland sits right at the base of the brain, protected by the skull from injury from even the dumbest male behaviors.

Right behind (and sometimes on top of) each testicle is the **epididymis**. This structure holds maturing sperm preparing for their journey. Their final launch from the epididymis is only an intermediate stage, however, as the sperm must then travel into the pelvis for final preparations. The epididymis is usually noticed by men only when they do self-examinations looking for testicle tumors. It may feel like a lump the first time someone notices it, but this is a normal structure and patients who notice it can be reassured that it belongs there. However, if you feel a lump, it is advisable to have it examined by a physician to determine whether it is safe or not.

The testicles are suspended precariously from each side of the abdomen by the **spermatic cords**—woven ropes of arteries, veins, muscles, nerves, and other tissues. The most important and strongest structure in the spermatic cord is the **vas deferens**. This structure carries sperm on the first part if its journey from the epididymis. It enters the abdomen through the *inguinal canal* (the *groin*) and heads toward the **prostate**. The vas deferens is the hard structure in the upper **scrotum** that feels like a matchstick. It is as sensitive as the testis in some men, so squeezing on it can be just as painful.

It makes sense that the testes wouldn't lie side by side, since the simple action of bringing the legs together could smash the testicles into each other. Instead, their unequal position allows them to slide right past each other when anything pushes them together. The left testis usually hangs a little lower than the right, at least in the northern hemisphere. No one knows why. If you know why, please spread the word.

The spermatic cords contain *cremasteric muscles* that are partially responsible for the "hang." Cold temperatures cause the cremasteric muscles to contract, pulling the testes up tightly against the body wall to keep them warm. Warm temperatures relax them, allowing the testicles to air cool. The *dartos muscles* of the scrotum assist in this temperature-mediated relocation.

The movement of the testicles with changes in temperature is based on their need to be a couple of degrees cooler than body temperature. Sperm cells form best just slightly below body temperature, which is why some people wear boxers instead of briefs when they're trying to achieve pregnancy. This is controversial, and it probably doesn't work. An excellent book on this topic is *Overcoming Male Infertility: Understanding Its Causes and Treatment* by Leslie R. Schover and Anthony Thomas, M.D.[1]

The testicles' need for a cooler environment is enigmatic. This is the only body process that requires a different temperature for its function in healthy conditions. The enigmatic part is that this makes it necessary for the testes, truly vital organs from the standpoint of preservation of the species, to be the only vital organs so vulnerable in their location. Despite this vulnerability, it is rare that someone loses both testicles other than at the hands of a surgeon or an adversary. Therefore, even if someone loses one testicle, it will usually cover the work of two, so the species is pretty safe.

(IN)FAMOUS TESTICLES: SOMETIMES YOU FEEL LIKE A NUT

Testicles don't have the exciting history of penises, but a few standouts are known. Both Hitler and Napoleon were said to have had one testis (each). This is usually due to a situation known as *undescended testis*, and is a result of abnormal fetal development. The testicles normally get their start inside the body cavity at the level of the kidneys during fetal development. As the body grows, they slowly descend until each one exits the body cavity through an *inguinal canal* (groin) on its way to the scrotum. This usually happens by the time the baby is delivered. If one or both testes are held up at any point along the way, they are called *undescended or cryptorchid* and should be surgically brought down into the scrotum during the first year or two of life. This situation is related to a higher risk of testis cancer and difficulties procreating, but it didn't contribute to the obnoxiousness of either Hitler or Napoleon.

On the way down, the testicles occasionally get lost as well. If they take a wrong turn, they can end up in either the abdominal wall or thigh.

Whether lost or just undescended, they are referred to as *ectopic* if they are anywhere other than their natural havens in the scrotum, and should be surgically redirected to the right spot while the owner is still in diapers.

The opposite condition—an extra testicle—is very rare. This is termed *polyorchidism* and is mainly found in anecdotal reports. The hundredth case in world medical literature was recently reported.[2]

Nine men with three testicles (each) were purportedly identified during conscription for World War II, although no one seems to know who was keeping a list. Probably as accurate was the exclamation of the lead male character in the movie *My Big Fat Greek Wedding,* who was tricked into blurting out that he had three testicles during a family gathering while trying to adapt to the Greek tongue of his fiancée.

A Guatemalan shaman named Don Pedro was known for having three testicles. The condition was identified during some horrible illness that the gods struck him with when he tried to avoid his sacred calling. While nursing him back to health, his mother found that he had three testicles. The urological revelation convinced Don Pedro and his family of his divine calling.

In reality, most men who believe they have an extra testicle actually have a fluid collection called a *spermatocele.* This collection of spermatic fluid can be differentiated from a third testicle by shining a penlight through it. If light shines through, it's just spermatic fluid and there is no alarm unless it gets too big to fit in the pants. Men often like the extra bulk that is noticeable through their jeans, so many will live with it and smile. That's fine as long as your physician confirms it is not a tumor.

ORCHIECTOMY

> If a male, perhaps due to natural defect or due to castration, is without [the two testicles], then he does not have ... this virile wind that erects the stem to its full strength. For that reason, the stem cannot become erect to plough woman like soil.
> —Hildegard of Bingen, twelfth century c.e.

Surgical removal of the testicles is called an *orchiectomy.* Historically, removal was mainly performed to punish men whose sexual practices offended someone, or to keep the young male opera singers in the soprano section instead of going through puberty and moving into the bass section.

These unfortunate vocalists were called the *castrati*, precursors of the androgynous singers popular during recent years.

Testicular cancer is a more appropriate indication for orchiectomy. This disease is the most common cause of solid (i.e., nonleukemia) tumors in young men. Therefore, all men below the age of forty-five should do monthly testicular self-exams to check for lumps within the substance of the testis. Timing this with a wife's breast exam is a good way to remember to do so monthly. The exam should be done during a warm shower so the scrotal contents are relaxed enough to feel any lumps.

It is important to differentiate between lumps within the testicle itself, which are usually malignant, versus lumps outside the testis, which are not. If uncertain, a urologist should perform an examination. He will try to determine if it is inside or outside the testis. This may involve shining a light through it as described above (a great trick to use at a Halloween party). If light shines through, it is just spermatic fluid and needs no treatment unless it is large enough to cause discomfort. If he can't tell, then an ultrasound is a noninvasive test that can readily detect the difference.

Men who have had undescended testes are at higher risk of testis cancer. This risk is not only in the affected testis, but in the other one as well. The reason the other testis is at risk is unclear, but it is probably due to whatever abnormality caused the one testis not to descend properly in the first place. This might have been a hormonal or genetic aberration, so it increases the likelihood the other testis will be abnormal due to the underlying problem and not necessarily to the fact that one doesn't descend.

Testicular cancer is described as the first true victory over cancer. Several high-profile young healthy athletes have beaten the disease, testifying to the near-universal success. It is rare for men to die of testicular cancer if treatments are given, so never avoid going to the doctor for fear of bad news.

The exemplum for surviving this disease is bicyclist Lance Armstrong. Armstrong had such advanced disease that it had even spread to his brain. Nevertheless, with modern treatments and his will not only to live, but also to live beyond anyone's imagination, he finished his treatment course and returned to the sport. After all that, he went on to win bicycling's premier event, the Tour de France, five times (so far). No sports comeback compares.

Unlike other cancers that have affected celebrities, there is not a single death in the past 30 years among the readily recognizable names. Olympian Scott Hamilton, baseball player John Kruk, and comedian Tom Green have all fully recovered. Alexandr Solzhenitsyn survived the Soviet health care system. Moreover, Hsing-Hsing, the world's most famous giant panda, did as well in the care of the veterinary team at the National Zoo.

Watching the made-for-television movie *Brian's Song* is the last time many American men admit to crying. Had Brian Piccolo of the Chicago Bears been diagnosed only a few years later, *Brian's Song* might have had a happy ending with the success of therapy currently available. (Interestingly, in the seventies the film didn't acknowledge the source of the protagonist's cancer. This taboo was gone by the year 2000, when comedian Tom Green's show on MTV gained ratings by celebrating the loss of his cancerous testis.)

The lesson is, testis cancer no longer has to be fatal or embarrassing, so do the self-exam and deal with it if you ever feel a lump.

A NOBEL EFFORT

Orchiectomy is also sometimes performed to treat prostate cancer. This sounds a little strange to remove the testicles instead of the cancerous gland, but makes sense when you realize that testosterone is the engine that drives the growth of prostate cancer. The first (and so far, only) urologist to earn the Nobel Prize was Dr. Charles B. Huggins. His prize-winning discovery in 1966 showed that protecting prostate cancer cells from the male hormone testosterone would slow their growth. Prior to that time, patients whose advanced cancers had spread were untreatable. Thereafter, Dr. Huggins' discovery allowed urologists to develop methods to block the growth factor of the cancer and yield significant results.

This was the first time anyone showed that cancer growth could be dependant on hormones. The concept subsequently led to the same type of discoveries regarding breast cancer in women. The management of both these diseases still depends on concepts that Dr. Huggins developed in the forties.

Dr. Huggins' discovery made two major contributions to urology. The first was to completely change our management of this previously untreatable disease. The second was to show the world that the young specialty of urology was on track to become a particularly respected branch of medicine.

We can now perform *medical castration* by injecting medications that block testosterone. The testicles are effectively turned off, so they can remain in place, albeit for cosmetic purposes only. These agents are very expensive, but very few men are willing to have the testicles physically removed in place of blocking them medically. A recent study in the *Journal of Urology* reported that men were willing to pay almost four hundred dollars a month to take these medications for the rest of their lives in order to avoid orchiectomy[3]—four hundred dollars a month for the ability to have nonfunctioning testicles in place. This attests to men's desire to maintain normal body image even in the face of cancer. Only one or two people ever see them (the man and his partner), but as one man told a friend, "They sure do dress a man up."

As mentioned, one testicle can usually do the work of two, so removal of only one of them will not result in enough of a decrease in testosterone to treat prostate cancer.

UNFRIENDLY ORCHIECTOMY: THE UNKINDEST CUT

Urological orchiectomy (surgically removing the testicles) is a recent phenomenon, but castration has a long history culturally. Somehow, it became known that removal of the testes made animals develop female characteristics. As early as 4000 B.C.E. the Neolithic tribes in Asia Minor domesticated dogs using castration. Early choirmasters used this to keep their young sopranos (castrati) singing in a high pitch well after puberty should have moved them to the tenor section.

Castration should be distinguished from orchiectomy, as the latter term means the removal of a testicle. In contrast, castration means that the hormones of *both* testicles are blocked, either medically or by orchiectomy of *both* testicles. Surgically removing one testicle will not effectively block hormone or sperm production.

In ancient times, harems needed men around for protection and other duties. The one duty not to be served by these men was prevented by orchiectomy. At least they thought so. As it turns out, many of these men could still have intercourse, since testicles aren't always required to have an erection. Since testosterone is key to **libido**, these men may not have sought or enjoyed intercourse as much as they would have preferred. Nevertheless, their female partners could be satisfied with no fear of a pregnancy conceived with someone other than their master, which would cost them their lives.

Orchiectomy has also been used for attitude readjustment. Sex offenders have occasionally received the treatment as a urological version of "an eye for an eye." An Arkansas man named Wayne Dumond was accused of raping a distant cousin of then-Governor Bill Clinton. Some friends of the young woman dished out some urological justice, removing Dumond's testicles. They ended up on the sheriff's desk as a warning to those who would consider such crimes in the jurisdiction. Where they are now, no one admits to. (Who would want them?)

Castration has been advocated as a means to control inappropriate or illegal sexual behaviors like rape or pedophilia. Babylonians around 2000 B.C.E. used it as punishment for adultery. However, the effect of orchiectomy on a man's ability to have intercourse is very unpredictable. Up to one-third of castrated men will continue to have normal function, while others will lose all sexual urges and functions (See "The role of hormones in the normal erection" in chapter 4). This makes its use as a deterrent for sex crimes unreliable and illogical. To date, nothing has proven to be medically or surgically effective to prevent criminals from committing such crimes.

SPERM: DNA BOMB WITH A TAIL

The main purpose evolutionarily for the testes is filling school bus seats, so it's not surprising they spend most of their time and energy producing sperm. Each testis can produce millions of sperm a day. Starting at around age twelve to fourteen, this translates into zillions of sperm a year, or a bajillion sperm in a typical seventy-seven-year life expectancy, give or take a few. About thirty to sixty million of these little DNA smart bombs are released every time an average man ejaculates, giving the egg little fighting chance of escape. When the nuns told you in high school that "it only takes once," it was with these odds in mind.

Sperm cells are remarkably similar among species. The sperm of the tiniest shrew is about the same size as that of a whale or elephant. Before the microscope was invented, sperm cells weren't visible at all. Then, in 1677, Antoni van Leeuwenhoek reported one of the first discoveries using a microscope when he found sperm cells in the ejaculate. Although using adequate modern equipment they look more like a tadpole, he thought he could see an entire human being small enough to be invisible to the naked eye within each sperm cell. He called these tiny microadults the *homunculus* and subsequently became known as the "Father of Sperm." As is often the case, the actual credit should have gone to one of van Leeuwenhoek's students, Ludwig Ham. Ludwig reportedly brought in a sample— unheard of in his day—to show the professor that he had found live creatures swimming in the cup using the microscope. All he got for his trouble was a footnote largely forgotten in medical history, while Professor van Leeuwenhoek became a legend.

SPERMATIC CORD: LIFELINE TO THE BODY

The *spermatic cord* suspends the testis from the abdomen. It exits the groin through the opening in the abdominal wall that the testis made during its descent to the scrotum. Hippocrates believed the testicles were attached to the penis through the spermatic cord like a system of pulleys. Damage to the cords would therefore render a man incapable of erecting the penis. Thus, he would be unable to achieve an erection following castration due to an absence of the counterweights required to pull on the cords.

If this opening doesn't close behind the escaping testis, an *inguinal hernia* results from the weakness created in the abdominal wall. A hernia is a weakening in any structure allowing things to push through. In the inguinal (groin) area, the intestines and other abdominal structures can push through the weakened muscle. About 25 percent of men will need hernia surgery during their lifetime to correct this weakness.

Rarely, the testis will twist on its cord and die. This condition, called *testicular torsion* (twisting), squeezes the blood vessels in the cord like wringing a towel. It results from a cord that is too long and loose, allowing the testis to spin around until blood flow is compromised. Testis cells are very fragile and can live for only a few hours without blood flow, so this is about the most urgent urological emergency that can occur.

The diagnosis of torsion is suspected by sudden onset of severe testicular pain in a male anywhere between puberty and middle age, usually on the younger end. An immediate trip to the emergency room is necessary. The physician may be able to *detorse* (untwist) it, but even so, the testes should both be secured into position once they have been shown capable of torsing. This operation, called *orchidopexy*, will prevent further damage from occurring.

VAS DEFERENS

The vas deferens carries sperm from the testicles into the pelvis. They empty into the **seminal vesicles** (see below) near the prostate, where they are stored for the final time. These small sperm highways are about the diameter of a matchstick. The ancient anatomists called this structure *vas*, which means "vein." They incorrectly believed it was a blood vessel to the testicle (obviously not tracing it up to find that it drains into the prostate instead of leading to the heart).

Until the late nineteenth century, male sterilization was assured only by orchiectomy. Unfortunately, not only did that stop sperm production, but also sometimes stopped **semen** production if it decreased the man's desire for intercourse. Later it was found that simply removing a segment of the vas deferens would stop sperm from making their way from the testicles into the semen. Thereafter the semen would look normal to the naked eye but would contain none of the little DNA bombs.

That operation is called **vasectomy.** Usually performed in the office setting using local anesthesia, one or two small incisions are made in the scrotum to remove a short segment of the vas deferens. Each end is sealed by the surgeon's method of choice and allowed to drop back into the scrotum. The procedure takes between three and sixty minutes, depending on a number of factors, including the patient's body habitus (build) and the experience and skill of the surgeon.

Three different methods are described to perform vasectomy. Most vasectomies are performed by the *classical* method, where separate incisions are made over each vas deferens using traditional surgical techniques. Dr. Li Shunqiang of China pioneered the *no-scalpel vasectomy* in the 1970s as an efficient way to meet the demand for mandatory sterilization in the world's most populous nation. Millions of men worldwide have benefited from this less invasive and faster alternative that removes a segment of each vas deferens through a small, single puncture in the scrotum.

Percutaneous vasectomy combines the best elements of both types. Using a version of the instruments developed for the no-scalpel vasectomy, a minimally invasive vasectomy is performed through two smaller incisions in a manner similar to a classical vasectomy.

Whichever method is chosen, vasectomy is by far the most reliable form of permanent birth control available. Compared to an annual pregnancy rate of about 8 percent for couples choosing the birth control pill, vasectomy fails in only one in several hundred cases. Even female tubal ligation fails ten times as often. (A discussion of birth control considerations is included in chapter 5.)

SCROTUM: UGLY WORD—UGLY STRUCTURE

The scrotum is the sac that contains spermatic cords and testes. The *dartos muscles* of the scrotum act with the *cremasteric muscles* of the spermatic cords to elevate or lower the testes to keep them at the right temperature. The wrinkles of the scrotum are due to these muscles being in various states of contraction. As they contract, the scrotal wall pulls up and thickens to warm the testes. As they relax, the scrotum thins and allows the testes to reach the right temperature as they drop away from the warmth of the body. As noted above, both Hitler and Napoleon were reported to each have a single testicle. As the defeat of each was attributed to attacking Russia in winter, one could wonder if their scrotal temperature controls were off.

The scrotum shares two characteristics with the eyelids. They are the only skin areas that contain no underlying fat, and they are the areas most prone to droop.

PROSTATE: THE SOUL OF UROLOGY

The center of the universe may be the penis for many men, but it's the prostate for most urologists. Although it has no role in an erection, no major male sexual function is ever very far removed from the prostate. This gland, about the size of a golf ball, sits wrapped around the urethra between the male bladder and penis. This strategic location makes it the Panama Canal of male anatomy. The Greek origin of the word *prostate* means "guardian," and nothing passes without going through its gates.

The real role of the prostate is to produce *semen*. After a man is beyond desire to reproduce, its main role is to keep doctors' offices full. Some of the reasons are discussed below.

PROSTATE PROBLEMS:
OBSTRUCTION AND INJUSTICE

The prostate gets blamed for more problems than El Niño. Culpability is sometimes fair, as when urination slows due to the enlarging gland squeezing around the **urethra** (*obstruction*). However, it's unfairly accused of being responsible for **erectile dysfunction** (the *injustice*). Yes, treatments for prostatic ailments can affect the nerves to the penis (see chapter

6), but the gland itself is an innocent bystander in regards to causing erectile dysfunction.

The reason it is blamed for erectile dysfunction is twofold. First, since there is an aura to the prostate due to its hidden location "down there," it is easy to let the imagination go wild on how harmful this evil little gland is. Second, erectile dysfunction often occurs in the same men who have prostate problems. As men age, they become more prone to all the conditions of maturity. However, prostate enlargement is no more responsible for erectile dysfunction than are other conditions of aging like baldness or gray hair. They just seem to all show up at the same time and in the same people. In addition, whereas the prostate was such a good friend when you were trying to have babies, now it just keeps you up at night and increases visits to the urologist.

Evidence of prostate enlargement starts with symptoms of urinary blockage or *obstruction*. The obstruction comes on slowly, so weakness in urinary stream may not be noticed at first. The initial signs may be when it takes longer to start the stream, especially in the morning when the bladder is stretched from filling all night. This, plus the fact the whole body is still a little sleepy, means the bladder muscle can't push as strongly against the mild blockage. Later in the day, its effects may be imperceptible.

As obstruction progresses, there may be a trip or two to the restroom in the middle of the night. It will also take longer to empty the bladder with a slower flow. You may notice a couple of guys at the ball game come and leave the urinals next to you before you finish your business. (Urologists tease about handing out business cards in the restrooms at ballgames to the guys who tie up the lines. Just remember to line up behind the young drunk guys, not behind the old drunk guys, and you'll be back in your seat before the first batter in the bottom of the inning.) These signs are moderate evidence of obstruction and may just be a nuisance that doesn't necessarily require treatment.

Later in the process, urinary frequency and an urgency to run to the bathroom indicate that the bladder is beginning to work excessively in order to push urine beyond the obstruction. You might miss the start of the next inning waiting for the bladder to empty. However, the frequency is sometimes due to incomplete emptying of the bladder. If it's still *half* full (because it only partially emptied during urination) as you leave the bathroom, you don't have as long until it is *completely* full and you need to void again. This is when treatment should probably not be further delayed. Several medications will relieve these symptoms, so most men will avoid surgery for this condition. Surgery to widen the channel through the prostate can be performed if medications aren't successful.

PROSTATITIS: NOT AS EVIL AS BELIEVED

Another prostatic diagnosis that gets blamed for the many ills of mankind is **prostatitis**. This is an inflammatory condition of the prostate that may be due to infection but is more commonly due simply to irritation or inflammation—sort of an arthritis of the prostate. Although some men really do have this inflammation, the diagnosis tends to be given as a catch-all for many symptoms that men have "down there." Therefore, if a man has symptoms anywhere between his belly button and his knees, the diagnosis of prostatitis may be inaccurately pinned on him.

Many patients and physicians believe prostatitis can cause either erectile dysfunction or **rapid** (or **premature**) **ejaculation**. However, there is no good reason to believe it contributes to either. The only exception to this is when the power of suggestion makes the patient believe it will cause sexual problems, as mental issues can contribute to either condition. If prostatitis could really cause these problems, then antibiotics should cure them. We know that is not the case.

Real symptoms of prostatitis include urinary difficulty or burning, along with pain in the "bottom." Perhaps the most significant symptom related to sexual activity is painful ejaculation. In that uncommon situation, prostatitis treatment can help. Otherwise, try to avoid the trap of blaming sexual problems on prostatitis in order to being thrown off-track.

PROSTATE CANCER

The prostate is the most common site for cancer in men. Fortunately, these cancers are usually treatable if detected early, so urologists advocate aggressive screening. That means a **PSA (Prostate Specific Antigen)** blood test and rectal examination every year after the age of fifty, stopping only when you get old enough that this usually slow-growing cancer is unlikely to cause a problem. This is around seventy to seventy-five, unless you have the genetic background to make it to a century or are an exceptional specimen. Men at risk of prostate cancer—including black men and those with a family history of prostate cancer—should begin screening five to ten years earlier. The tricky part is that some prostate cancers can be more aggressive, so assumptions that any given case will be indolent are hazardous.

PSA is a chemical produced by the prostate that turns semen into a more liquefied form several minutes after ejaculation. By that time, enough sperm have started their journey toward the egg that they don't need to be held together in the thicker form.

After procreating is completed, PSA really doesn't do anything. Scientists didn't even discover it until the 1970s. For the first couple of decades after discovery, the molecule was a simple curiosity. Then we found that PSA was released into the blood stream in higher amounts in certain disease states of the prostate, cancer being the one of obvious interest. Our understanding of PSA is still in the works, but we know that it is the best screening tool available at this time to detect prostate cancer.

The PSA blood test should be combined with a rectal examination in order to optimize the early detection of prostate cancer. Men are usually more open to a blood test like PSA than to a rectal exam. This reticence is understandable. However, up to one fourth of all men with prostate cancer will have a normal PSA, so the exam must complement the PSA in order to screen adequately. If one or the other is omitted, many cases of cancer will go undetected, perhaps until it's too late.

PROSTATE BIOPSY: IT DOESN'T HAVE TO HURT

When prostate cancer is suspected—based on an elevated PSA or an abnormal rectal examination—a **biopsy** is required to confirm or rule out the diagnosis. A biopsy is an office-based procedure to obtain tissue samples from the prostate for pathological interpretation. The typical way this is performed is by placing an *ultrasound probe*, shaped like an examining finger, into the rectum to visualize the prostate. This allows a needle to take six to twenty-four small cores of prostate tissue.

Sound painful? Well, it used to be because we didn't know how to anesthetize the prostate. However, recent advances have allowed us to inject a local anesthetic into the nerves entering the prostate (identified by Dr. Patrick Walsh as described in chapter 2), thereby virtually eliminating all pain. Therefore, don't be nervous about having a prostate biopsy if your urologist recommends one, as long as you will receive a local anesthetic. If your urologist doesn't use local anesthesia, ask him to try it. Its success is now irrefutable, so it doesn't have to hurt anymore.

PSA SCREENING: THE CONTROVERSY

PSA testing is actually a little controversial. Some opponents of early detection believe that we are overdiagnosing prostate cancer by such rigorous testing. They suggest that if we'd just leave well enough alone, we would save many men what they think are unnecessary biopsies, X rays, surgery, or other treatments. This is based on the rationale that prostate cancer will often be a slow-growing disease. Therefore, if a man has a limited life expectancy anyway, maybe he will die of something else first.

That is true. If a man has a life expectancy of less than ten years, prostate cancer is unlikely to cause his early demise. However, if his life expectancy is greater than ten years, undiagnosed and untreated prostate cancer could make him one of 31,500 American men who die of the disease each year. Therefore, let's not make blanket statements that all men or no men should be screened for prostate cancer. Let's just say that men old enough to have prostate cancer, but young and healthy enough to expect at least ten more years before dying of natural causes, should undergo this easy screening test. As noted, the age to begin testing is about fifty years old for most men, but forty to forty-five for men at risk, namely black men and men with a family history of the disease.

Since this is controversial, most men should discuss this with their own primary care physician or urologist in order to make an informed decision about early detection of prostate cancer.

A TOMATO A DAY KEEPS THE UROLOGIST AWAY

Cancer prevention is a hot topic. Although many things have been advocated without evidence, we do have reason to believe that there are some lifestyle changes that can lessen the chance of developing prostate cancer.

We know that men who eat a low-fat diet are less likely to develop prostate cancer. The type of fat consumed has been controversial, but there is no clear evidence that the "Got Cancer?" ads are accurate in their assertion that consuming milk or other substances containing animal fats causes prostate cancer. Studies that may elucidate this are ongoing.

Asian men have a diet low in fat as well as high in soy-based products. This is thought to contribute to their lower incidence of prostate cancer. Therefore adding soy proteins to a healthy diet can't hurt.

Vitamin E and *selenium* have been shown possibly to decrease the chance of developing several types of cancer, including prostate cancer. There is enough evidence that many urologists routinely recommend their supplementation, as long as patients stick to maximum recommended doses.[4] This is especially important with selenium, which can be toxic in excessive doses.

In addition, a large multi-institutional trial is currently in process to find out whether men who take these two supplements will have less incidence of prostate cancer down the road. This trial is creatively named SELECT, meaning the **SEL**enium and Vitamin **E** Cancer prevention Trial. If you have interest in participating, call 1-800-422-6237 (1-800-4-CANCER). The trial is open to any man above the age of fifty and black men above the age of forty-five (due to the increased cancer risk in this group).

Another prevention trial involved *finasteride*, a medication that blocks testosterone from being converted to its active form in cells. Finasteride is marketed already as two different prescription drugs. The first is the stronger, 5-milligram size called *Proscar*, which is used to shrink an enlarged prostate. The 1-milligram size of the identical chemical is marketed as *Propecia*, familiar as the once-a-day pill prescribed for male pattern baldness. This study was closed in 2003 when researchers found that the risk of prostate cancer was reduced by 25 percent when taking finasteride. However, the men who developed cancer appeared to have more aggressive disease, so we still can't define the role of finasteride in prevention.

The only other thing that we have good reason to believe lessens the risk of prostate cancer is a diet high in tomatoes. They contain *lycopene*, an *antioxidant* that is released in high quantities when tomatoes are cooked. Antioxidants are chemicals that theoretically scavenge up *free radicals*, chemical byproducts that are believed to cause many cases of cancer. Men eating a diet high in tomato products, especially when cooked, seem to be less likely to develop prostate cancer.[5] In light of all this information, consider taking vitamin E and selenium, or going onto the SELECT trial. Try to lean toward a diet high in soy and low in fat. When ordering dinner, choose the red sauce instead of the white every time.

SEMINAL VESICLES

The seminal vesicles are sacs that sit behind the bladder, attached to the prostate. Over half of the ejaculate is produced by these hidden secondary sex glands of which few people have ever heard. Each vas deferens joins the ducts from the seminal vesicles in a joint duct called the *ejaculatory duct.* During an **ejaculation**, muscle contractions push semen down the ejaculatory duct, through the prostate, and out to do its work if things are working properly. (This process is covered in chapter 5.) Otherwise, the seminal vesicles may be the most boring organs in the body.

SEMEN

It wasn't until 1779, three years after American independence from England, that Lazzaro Spallanzani of Italy demonstrated that semen was produced in the secondary sex organs and was necessary for fertilization. Prior to that time, it was widely accepted that semen was just a product of the entire body that was meant for the pleasure of sexual intercourse.

The ejaculate normally consists of two to six cubic centimeters of semen. Most people assume this is mostly sperm, but the little tadpoles actually form less than 1 percent of this fluid. Most of semen comes from the seminal vesicles, the prostate, and smaller glands. It is high in fructose (a sugar usually found in fruit), potassium, zinc, citric acid, and a host of enzymes. This relatively massive amount of sugar is the nourishment required to support the sperm on its happy journey. It must swim the equivalent of thirty miles compared to its body size, then beat out about forty to sixty million other microscopic Don Juans for the right to dig into the egg, fertilize its own DNA packet, and then never again escape. A Pyrrhic victory is the best it can hope for.

In addition to these sugars for the little guys to snack on during the journey are other chemicals that make the route more hospitable. The ejaculate is released as a thick gel so that it does not run immediately out of the **vagina**. This allows the sperm time to begin their trek toward the egg without slipping right back out. After a few minutes, the gel spontaneously liquefies to facilitate further upwards migration. One of the main chemicals causing this liquefaction is PSA. This is the same chemical described above that is used to screen for prostate cancer.

Rock music legend has it that the group 10 CC chose its name based on the volume of an ejaculation. That overestimates the reality by about double. Rumors of other rock stars and seminal volumes are pretty wild, but also probably just that—rumors. In contrast, as noted earlier, a boar reportedly ejaculates up to a liter of semen!

KEY POINTS

- The secondary sex organs mainly produce semen and mobilize it in a concerted effort to perpetuate the species.
- The effect of castration on erections is unpredictable, but it will always render a man sterile (incapable of fathering children) if both testicles are removed.
- All men over the age of fifty (and black men over the age of forty-five) should be screened for early detection of prostate cancer by using a PSA blood test and a rectal examination annually.

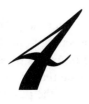

The Normal Erection
What Could Go Wrong?

[Man] has imagined a heaven, and has left entirely out of it the supremest [*sic*] of all his delights, the one ecstasy that stands first and foremost in the heart of every individual of his race—and ours—sexual intercourse!

—Mark Twain, *Letters from the Earth*, written 1909

*D*efining "normal" when the topic is sex may not be possible. Typical behavior, frequency, and variety depend on the people involved. Still, we can describe what happens to the penis during a normal erection.

An erection occurs when blood fills the corpora cavernosae (see chapter 2) with enough pressure to cause rigidity. This occurs when inflow exceeds outflow to a pressure of about 100 mm mercury. In this chapter we will describe the elements that are required for an erection, whereas the following chapter will tackle the bigger questions of how people normally use one.

ERECTIONS THROUGHOUT HISTORY

"When the man becomes inflamed with lust and desire, blood rushes into the male member and causes it to become erect."

—Ambrose Pare, 1585

Our understanding of how an erection occurs has changed over the years. Aristotle believed that nerve branches carried "spirit and energy" to the penis, which caused it to inflate with air. The observance of excess penile blood in hanged men allowed Leonardo da Vinci to cast aside the air-erection theory. Based on this work, Ambrose Pare in 1585 wrote the passage above, qualifying him to be considered the first romance novelist.

In 1573, the Italian anatomist Varolio discovered the *bulbocavernosus* and *ischiocavernosus muscles* around the root of the penis. The only possible conclusion was that these muscles tightened to produce an erection. Unable to test the theory in a real person (who would want an incision made during an erection?), the idea persisted for centuries.

The early twentieth century brought several variations of a theory that "polsters" were magical, miniscule anatomical parts that caused the normal erection. These polsters were supposed to be small hydraulic pumps that miraculously knew when to open and close to allow adequate filling. This theory fell into disfavor when no one could actually find "polsters" in any dissection, microscopically, or otherwise.

We now know the process is actually fairly straightforward: the bottom line is that the arteries must let in more blood than the veins let out for adequate pressure to build. When this blood is temporarily trapped under pressure, the results are uplifting.

NO WAY: NITRIC OXIDE PAVES THE WAY

The chemical, called a *neurotransmitter*, that is central to the erection process is **nitric oxide** (ironically abbreviated **NO**). Nitric oxide is more commonly known to most people as an air pollutant. It is often confused with nitrous oxide, more appropriately abbreviated N_2O, which is an anesthetic gas.

The work leading up to the discovery that NO is key to erections began in the seventies. Three different American researchers began studying arterial dilation, when the wisest of them identified NO as the chemical that signaled to smooth muscles in arterial walls to relax. It was only a matter of time before a connection to erections was made.

The connection was made when Dr. Jacob Rajfer, professor of urology at the UCLA School of Medicine, was stuck on the freight elevator at the medical school in late 1988. "It was a very slow elevator with doors that stay open too long. We'd been complaining about it for years," he remembers. As is common among research physicians, he had been putting a lot of thought into a clinical question regarding his research interest in vascular smooth muscle. He had been trying to figure out how the vascular smooth muscle in the penis was involved in an erection when he looked through the slowly closing doors of the elevator and saw the sign to the Vascular Smooth Muscle Lab, a completely separate department from urology. "I put out my hand to stop it," he recalls. "It was totally serendipitous."[1]

Dr. Rajfer went into the lab for the first time and set up a meeting with the head of the lab, Dr. Louis Ignarro, who had already begun work on the idea. Once they connected the research dots, it was a matter of time until scientists at Pfizer were able to capitalize on their findings with the discovery of Viagra. The rest is erection history. The efforts of Dr. Ignarro, along with pharmacologists Robert F. Furchgott and Ferid Murad, were rewarded with almost a million dollars in 1998, when they were named the winners of the Nobel Prize in Medicine.

NO was also named "Molecule of the Year" by *Science* magazine in 1992 for its involvement in so many different actions. Although it is also involved in processes as varied as preventing bone loss (?) to dilating the penile blood vessels, it's pretty obvious which action grabbed the attention of the Nobel committee. It can't be a coincidence that they won the Nobel Prize the year Viagra hit the market.

The real coincidence is that the committee awarded the Nobel Prize for research that began when Dr. Murad tried to find out how nitroglycerin affects blood vessels. Ironically, Swedish industrialist Alfred Nobel, namesake of the prize, refused to take nitroglycerin for his heart condition because it gave him headaches. Instead, he used nitroglycerin to invent TNT, which provided the fortune that still funds these prizes. Interestingly, taking nitroglycerin would have prevented Mr. Nobel from using Viagra, as the combination of these two drugs is contraindicated and *can be fatal.*

Sexual stimulation triggers the release of nitric oxide from nerve endings. It opens the penile arteries so blood rushes in. The **sinusoids**, which are spaces inside the penis that allow blood to build up under pressure, fill up as a result. As these sinusoids fill, they help compress the veins leading out of the penis, thereby forcing the pressure inside the corpora cavernosae to reach heights sufficient to stand up straight. This pressure, over 100 mm mercury, is not enough to inflate a tire, but not bad.

PHYSICAL REQUIREMENTS
FOR A NORMAL ERECTION

This is the monstruosity in love, lady—that the will is infinite and
the execution confined; that the desire is boundless and the act a
slave to limit.
　　　　　　—William Shakespeare, *Troilus and Cressida*, act 5, scene 2

Obviously, the penis must be served by normal supply lines for all this to
work. Most important are arteries to carry blood in and veins to control its
escape. Also required for a trouble-free, natural erection are normal nerves
to signal the hard drive to boot up, normal hormones (mainly to make you
interested), and a psyche that doesn't flood the system with "abort" mes-
sages before the job is done.

The stimulation to start these events can come from a number of different origins. The ones we're most familiar with are obvious. However,
chemicals injected into the penis can override all other signals. (Chapter 13
describes how this can be used to effectively treat difficult cases of erectile
dysfunction.)

Another situation of erection occurring without sexual stimulation
occurs during sleep, yielding the morning erections every man knows
about. The body naturally sends randomly timed signals to cause erections
that peak during rapid eye movement (REM) sleep. These are responsible
for the pup tent first experienced in boyhood. REM sleep is the deepest
phase of sleep, occurring mainly toward morning, which explains why
these erections are usually noticed upon awakening. The presence of these
nocturnal erections is a useful diagnostic clue, as discussed in chapter 7.

Any male who was called to the chalkboard in junior high school
knows spontaneous erections occur with unpredictable regularity in adolescents, sometimes with no more stimulation than a good gust of wind. These
diminish greatly after the **testosterone** storm of puberty abates. Men often
worry when these spontaneous erections become less frequent, but this
change as men age is natural. An erection noticeable to the algebra class is
a minor embarrassment, but an erection in front of a board meeting would
just be too much. No one should worry about an absence of erections
during the normal daily routine as long as they appear on demand when the
day is done.

Men with spinal cord injuries and certain other neurological conditions
can have reflex erections unrelated to external stimuli. This is a reflex based

on nerve activity going from the penis to spinal cord and back. The timing of this rarely correlates with opportunity, but with a little luck (or, more likely, with some urological assistance) might culminate in **orgasm**, **ejaculation**, and offspring if desired.

ONCE THE SIGNAL IS RECEIVED

Whatever the source of the signals, once the stimulation reaches the penis, a cascade develops. Nitric oxide naturally relaxes the smooth muscles of the penile arteries, allowing more blood to flow in. The veins going out of the penis close down at the same time, trapping blood inside and causing a buildup of pressure. As the pressure starts to mount, these veins are compressed against the **tunica albuginea** (see chapter 2) so pressure rises rapidly, as does the penis.

A breakdown in either inflow or outflow leads to failure. This occurs when either inflow becomes inadequate or outflow exceeds inflow. Troubles with inflow can occur at any point along the blood supply to the penis, but the common denominator among most of the causes of **erectile dysfunction** is that not enough blood gets to its destination. If that occurs, an erection may not.

Although it sounds appealing to think a blockage can be identified and opened up or bypassed in a manner similar to treating coronary artery disease (hardening of the arteries of the heart), success is rarely possible for erectile dysfunction using similar techniques. This is because the arteries to the penis are tiny to begin with. It's usually just a manner of narrowing through extended lengths of those arteries. (This is described in more detail in chapter 15.)

Problems with outflow, called **venous insufficiency**, are probably underestimated. Surgery to tie these veins off is sometimes used, but more commonly, a **constriction ring** is the answer (as discussed in chapter 11).

Interestingly, during erection there is very little actual blood flow. The blood coming in and going out are in balance, so the pressure stays high enough to keep the penis rigid as long as they remain in balance.

THE ROLE OF HORMONES
IN THE NORMAL ERECTION

The diagnosis of prostate cancer came as a shock to Mark, a fifty-three-year-old photographer, and his wife Kelly. They had one of the best marriages imaginable, clearly in love after twenty years. Kelly was a striking woman who could pass for a college student even in her forties.

Unfortunately, the cancer was already advanced before detection, so a cure was not possible. The treatment for advanced prostate cancer involves blocking the male hormone, *testosterone*, as described in chapter 3. Mark chose to block testosterone using a chemical injection that shuts down testicular production.

They were sexually active at least three times a week prior to his diagnosis, and this was clearly an important part of their relationship. During a frank discussion of the likelihood this treatment could make it difficult for Mark to have natural erections, they both agreed quickly that slowing the progression of the cancer was priority number one. Kelly's statement was, "I can't have sex with him if he's dead, either." The first injection was given during that visit, and he was scheduled for a second injection three months later. They left stating a plan to be as sexually active as they could be, for as long as they could, and said they would call when he needed treatment for inevitable erectile dysfunction.

There was no call prior to the follow-up visit three months later. The only complaint from either partner at that time was fatigue. They were worn out from the daily intercourse, and had voluntarily pared back because both were worn out. The only thing either of them had noticed was that Mark's interest was waning, but probably more due to the grueling sexual pace they were on than due to any true physical or mental changes.

Mark and Kelly moved out of state about a year after the treatments began, having returned to a more sustainable intercourse frequency of two or three times a week. This was more than Mark really required, but just right for Kelly. His PSA blood test, used to monitor the cancer, did not detect cancer, indicating an excellent response. They declined an offer for a Viagra prescription.

Until recently, it was believed that the only physical cause of impotence was related to low levels of testosterone, the male sex hormone. This condition is called **hypogonadism**, which means the gonadal production of testosterone is low ("hypo-").

The assumption that hypogonadism causes impotence made plenty of sense; everyone knows men without testicles (eunuchs) can't have erections, right?

Wrong. Eunuchs were chosen to protect harems, wives, or other females throughout history because they couldn't have sex. However, as noted earlier, the eunuchs often actually were able to have plenty of erections. Therefore, they were often meeting the sexual needs of the females they were charged with protecting—a dirty little secret through the ages. The females never got pregnant since these eunuchs didn't produce sperm (although they did **ejaculate**). That protected the participants—and the truth about the role of testosterone in erections—from discovery. It clearly demonstrates that testosterone is not crucial to erections, but it doesn't answer the exact role that this male hormone plays.

It appears that the most significant role testosterone plays in erections is in **libido**. Libido refers to sexual desire, not performance. A person with a large libido has significant desire or thoughts about sex. This is different from actually acting on those desires. Many men with erectile dysfunction have plenty of libido—they want sex but can't have it, at least not as often or as well as they desire. In fact, if their libido were less, the erectile dysfunction wouldn't be as great a concern since they wouldn't desire what they couldn't have (unless their partner's libido was the issue, which is sometimes the case). For this reason, men with low testosterone frequently don't complain, since they may not miss what they are missing out on. Many of these men are walking around perfectly happy in their state of decreasing libido, as long as their libido aligns somewhat with that of their partners.

In the situation of a man treated for prostate cancer by blocking testosterone, he would have the same level of testosterone that a castrated man would have—almost none. So why would he still have sexual desire to the level he did? Because libido involves many things, only one of which is testosterone. It also involves multifaceted aspects of relationships and sexual viewpoint—a pretty complex interaction. In a relationship where the man values the closeness of intercourse with his partner, he may retain his libido. In addition, he may be committed to meeting his mate's sexual needs.

Although relationship factors frequently contribute to erectile dysfunction, relationship factors can also overcome physical issues such as hypogonadism.

ORGASM: THE ULTIMATE GOAL?

An orgasm is the pleasurable event that occurs at the peak of sexual excitement. For women, it is a purely neurological occurrence involving a surge in output of the *parasympathetic* and *somatic nervous systems*. For men, this surge in neurological output is evidenced by contractions in the pelvic muscles and the forced ejaculation of **semen**. For women, the pleasurable sensations are apparently identical to those in men, but they lack the visible confirmation of ejaculation.

Masters and Johnson described four phases of the **sexual response cycle** for men and women. The first phase is *excitement*, which can last from minutes to hours. This encompasses everything from the emotions felt during dinner and conversation, to the swelling of the penis or **clitoris** during early phases of foreplay. The *excitement* phase is followed by a *plateau* in which stimulation is maximally sustainable. For men, this phase includes most of the duration the penis is erect. In contrast, women may reach *plateau* during foreplay, but also may not reach this phase until well after penetration.

The peak of sexual excitement occurs in the third phase, *orgasm*. The first thing men experience is **emission** of semen into the posterior **urethra,** giving them an intensely pleasurable sense that orgasm is inevitable. Once this occurs, some men can prolong the duration for a few seconds, but there is no holding back. Ejaculation of semen from the urethra is the usual obvious outcome. Women don't exhibit emission or ejaculation, but have the same feelings of inevitability. They experience a rhythmic contraction of the pelvic muscles and uterus during orgasm.

The final phase is a period of *resolution*, marked by a general sense of well being, enhanced intimacy, and fatigue. During the resolution phase, further genital stimulation is actually unpleasant instead of pleasurable. This is called the **refractory period**. Men lose the erection during this phase and are unable to have another orgasm until the refractory period ends.

Younger men have a short refractory period, lasting just minutes in some. However, the refractory period extends with aging, a fact that can become distressing to men who formerly could regain an erection while their partner was still aroused. With an increasing refractory period, he may be unable to return to the ballgame before she loses interest.

Authorities disagree on whether women normally have a refractory period, but clearly there is usually a period following orgasm in some women when further stimulation is "too much." This period is shorter in women than in men, so many women can achieve *multiple orgasms* during a single sexual encounter, while their male partners must settle for one.

As mentioned, orgasm can be broken down into two parts in the male. Emission is the release of semen into the urethra. The word *ejaculation* comes from the Latin word meaning "to throw a dart." Therefore, an ejaculation is the physical expulsion of semen from the urethra. This fluid has nothing to do with sexual enjoyment of either partner, so the absence of seminal fluid is only a problem if reproduction is desired.

Sometimes there is no expulsion of semen. This is called either **anejaculation** (an absence of semen), or **retrograde ejaculation**. Retrograde ejaculation occurs when the semen gets lost on the way out and turns into the bladder instead of coming out the urethra. Some medications like Flomax and Cardura cause this by relaxing the bladder neck. Since fluid will find the route of least resistance, it simply runs into the bladder and is expelled on the next void. Unless the patient wishes to father children this causes no concern. If he does, he will need reproductive assistance from an infertility specialist. This is different from **anorgasmia**, which is the situation where the man never reaches climax at all. This can be due to hormonal, physical, or psychological reasons.

Following a **TURP (transurethral resection of the prostate)** operation for **prostate** enlargement, the opening from the prostate into the bladder is enlarged, which also results in retrograde ejaculation. Following **radical prostatectomy** for cancer, there is not even an emission of semen. This is because all connection to the urethra is removed during this operation. These men can still enjoy a normal orgasm (the pleasurable feeling); they just don't have emission or ejaculation.

KEY POINTS

- An erection requires blood flowing into the penis at a rate high enough to overcome outflow. When trapped under adequate pressure, an erection occurs.
- The stimulus for a normal erection may be from sexual stimulation but may also occur from neurological signals during waking or sleeping hours.
- Spontaneous erections decrease with age. This should cause no concern as long as erections continue to occur during appropriate times.
- The role of testosterone in erections is complex, but it is mainly involved in maintaining libido.

- Orgasm is the pleasurable sensation associated with intense sexual stimulation. In men it is usually, but not always, accompanied by emission of semen into the urethra and a subsequent ejaculation of that semen. The same sensation occurs in women but without emission or ejaculation.
- Alfred Nobel refused to take nitroglycerin for his heart condition but instead used it to invent dynamite. He ironically used the resulting fortune to fund the peace prize that bears his name. The discovery of nitric oxide that eventually led to the development of Viagra for erectile dysfunction won the Nobel Prize. Just like Alfred Nobel, men who take Viagra should refuse to take nitroglycerin since the combination can be lethal. No one knows whether Alfred Nobel had erectile dysfunction.

5 Who Are Those People on Television?

Normal Sexual Function

Sex is a part of life. It can be fine and full and very beautiful. It can be painful, restricting, and shameful. Like every other source of power, it must be harnessed or it runs wild and becomes destructive. Electricity wired into your home will light your house, cook your meals, warm your feet, and perform all kinds of miracles. Left unleashed, as lightning, it can destroy everything you care about in one burning holocaust. So it is with sex.
        —Evelyn Millis Duvall, *Love and the Facts of Life*, 1967

*W*atching television gives an interesting view of sexual behavior. One would think that most adults spend a majority of their waking time and energy pursuing or enjoying sexual activity with a succession of multiple partners. These partners seldom get pregnant or catch sexually transmitted diseases. That doesn't sound like my neighborhood, so what is the truth about what's going on sexually out there? We will now explore what little is known about sexual norms, as well as other related issues regarding sexual behavior.

HOW OFTEN IS "NORMAL"?

> The wise physicians have stated that one in a thousand dies from
> other illnesses and the [remaining 999 in the thousand] from
> excessive sexual intercourse.
> —Moses ben Maimon (Maimonides), 1135–1204 C.E.

A psychologist friend mentioned a couple she was counseling regarding a disparity in libido. Ellen was not averse to sex, and in proper frequency actually enjoyed it. Earlier in their marriage, she and her husband Frank had intercourse more frequently, but after going through menopause, she wanted to slow down a bit.

Frank wasn't interested in slowing down and wanted things to remain just the same way as when they were as newlyweds forty-five years earlier. This scenario is common, so the story didn't seem too remarkable. The only reason they involved me was because erections were starting to take a little more stimulation, and Ellen wasn't motivated to do the extra work required. "What are his expectations?" I asked.

That's when it came out that this couple of septuagenarians continued to attempt intercourse five times every day. With the refractory period between erections getting longer, one or two of the sexual escapades had to occur during hours normally devoted to sleep. Frank actually set the alarm for 5 A.M. in order to get in the last scheduled union before the sunrise restarted the process. Their family physician had scheduled counseling because he felt the demands placed on Ellen were intolerable.

Based on her plea for a respite, he had instructed Frank that interrupting Ellen's sleep was unacceptable. A clear directive was laid down that Ellen was not to be awakened to perform what Frank considered her wifely duties. "You must wait until morning before making any advances," he was warned. In order to leave no room for interpretation, Frank was told that the alarm, normally set for 6:30, was not to be disturbed.

The following morning, Ellen awoke to find Frank standing over the bed, grinning and looking back and forth between Ellen and the alarm clock. Six twenty-three flashed in big red letters. Frank was poised.

The ideal frequency and timing of sexual activity is different for all persons. The axiom often heard is that men think of sex every eight seconds; their mind is just wandering between those eight-second intervals. Clearly, not even Frank could perform every eight seconds. Sometimes men may truly desire sex just because "it's been too long."

So, how long is "too long"? It depends upon whom you ask. Some people will be content never to have intercourse, whereas some will be dissatisfied if they do not have intercourse several times daily. Few would take it to the extremes of Frank, however. It was only after some intensive counseling that Frank became more realistic. Interestingly, the marriage was solid in every other way, so once his attitude was readjusted, they resumed a relationship satisfactory to both.

SEXUAL FREQUENCY SURVEYS: NO HELP

> The indulgence of sexual intercourse is one of the requirements for the maintenance of health, providing that there should be adequate abstinence between periods of indulgence, so that no noticeable enfeeblement or weakness ensue.
>
> —Maimonides

Statistics quoted on sexual surveys should be interpreted cautiously. First, these surveys have to assume that people will tell the truth. However, just as Kinsey found that men exaggerate about the size of their penises, we have to assume they aren't entirely truthful about sexual behavior. Second, it is unreasonable to think that an average would be meaningful. Averaging the number of sexual encounters of someone like Frank with the frequency of someone celibate would give a number that wasn't representative of either one of them, and sure wouldn't be representative of the population at large. Therefore, the averages are not a target that adults should shoot for, but rather a reference to shed a little light on what is really happening out there.

Since the Kinsey study performed in the mid-twentieth century, Americans appear to have increased their sexual behavior substantially. Most recently, studies indicate that American adults average a little over one sexual episode a week.[1] That number can be misleading, however, as the younger people in these surveys may have sex three to four times a week, while one in five adults at any given point in time *never* has sex. Between the ages of thirty-six and forty-five, the frequency of sexual activity has risen from seventy-five times a year to ninety-nine. That's an extra evening of romance every other week!

In the media, single people have most of the sex. Sexual behavior studies show that the opposite is true in the real world, with married people having much more frequent intercourse. Interestingly, people with children are also more sexually active than those without. And yes, this persists even *after* the children are conceived.

Those who work longer schedules use their free time more wisely than coworkers who don't put in the hours. It seems they also put in more effort in the bedroom and enjoy more active sex lives than their less energetic colleagues. Distressingly, greater levels of education are associated with less frequent sexual activity.

Certain lifestyles seem to be related to sexual activity, but sometimes unpredictably so. Jazz fans are more active than those who listen to hard rock. Paradoxically, both gun owners and liberals do fairly well sexually. Perhaps conservatism inhibits sexual activity unless you wield a big gun.

Religious differences can be pronounced. Jews and agnostics are more sexually active than Christians are. Catholics do okay, but Lutherans and Presbyterians aren't averaging their fair shares.

Regarding age, the patterns are predictable. Whereas almost all younger married people are sexually active, many senior citizens are never sexually active. It is estimated that 8 percent of senior citizens account for 85 percent of all elderly sexual activity. Obviously, averages in the older group are therefore meaningless.

SEX IS GOOD—AND GOOD FOR YOU

> As for a moderate commerce with the other sex, far from enfeebling nature, it preserves her in a right state: it was intended in our construction; and is required by our constitution.
>
> —John Hill, 1771

People who score more often also rate high scores on measures of happiness. In all demographic groups, sexually active adults are happier and healthier than those who are not. This begs the question of whether sex makes one happy, or whether being happy causes one to engage in sex more frequently. In all likelihood the two go hand in hand—coexistent instead of causative.

In addition, physical health is promoted by sexual activity. Recent studies have shown that frequency of sexual intercourse is inversely related to death rates in both men and women, but its exact role was different between the sexes.[2] The quantity (frequency) of intercourse was more important for longevity in men, while the quality of the sexual relationship was paramount for women's longevity.

This health benefit was actually more pronounced in women. If women enjoy intercourse, it has a positive health benefit. If they don't, but simply go through the motions to meet the frequency needs of a partner, there may be no health benefit. (Therefore, a healthy sexual relationship will attempt to meet the frequency needs of the man, while supplying the quality required for the woman.)

A recent study from Wales published in the *British Medical Journal* looked at the role of **orgasm** on health. Men were half as likely to die if they had over one hundred orgasms a year.[3] *Therefore*, even if you don't feel like it, try your best to have intercourse twice a week. If you have to miss a few reruns to achieve that goal, so be it. Your longevity is worth it.

SO, WHAT FREQUENCY IS RIGHT FOR ME?

Sex is like money. Only too much is enough.

—John Updike, 1968

Kent was disconsolate. Although he always found sex with his wife Alicia to be great, a discussion with fellow junior faculty members at the engineering department party left him feeling woefully inadequate. Before that party, he was satisfied with their sharing of intercourse two or three times weekly (except at semester's end, when both were short of free time), even as they approached their fifth wedding anniversary.

However, the stories told by his coworkers at the party made it clear that Kent and Alicia weren't keeping up with their colleagues. Randy was a newlywed who claimed that most days began and ended with an hour or more of lovemaking with his young bride. Dave had a live-in relationship with a psychology graduate student and boasted that they rarely missed an opportunity for romance. They made love almost every time they saw each other. Worst of all, the single Pierre seemed to have a new partner on a regular basis. He savored taunting the committed men in the department with hints of his conquests. Kent could only listen and hope that no one made him acknowledge that he made love to his wife only two or three times a week. It would be too embarrassing.

Kent would have been much less embarrassed had he known the truth.

Randy was indeed making love a little more often than Kent, but only because he was newly married. Within months, he and his wife had settled into a routine not unlike that of Kent and Alicia. Dave honestly reported that he and his graduate student roommate never wasted an opportunity. What he didn't elucidate was that their schedules overlapped about once a week, if they were lucky. The biggest exaggeration had come from Pierre. Indeed, he floated in and out of several brief sexual relationships, which usually were nothing more than one-night stands. However, about six nights a week Pierre slept alone. Had Kent only been able to ignore the bragging of the others, he would have realized that his sex life was not only satisfying to both him and Alicia, but was one of the healthiest and happiest of anyone he knew.

The Talmud recommends intercourse somewhere between daily and monthly, depending on the stage and standing in life of the man. It has been written that Mohammed recommended regular intercourse. Jesus apparently left it up to the flock to decide. The bottom line is that there is no universal normal frequency of intercourse.

Psychologically, the right amount of sex is that which makes both partners happy. Since total agreement between partners is unlikely, most couples have to work out a compromise. Effective communication between partners is the most likely way for them to both feel their position is represented fairly.

Physically, frequency of intercourse is limited in women and younger men only by free time, energy, and opportunity. However, the **refractory period** following orgasm puts limits on a man as he matures. Young men may be able to regain an erection within minutes of **ejaculation**, but the time required to recover increases with age. From *minutes* in the twenties, this time can be measured in *hours* by the fifties, and in *days* in the later decades.

This natural change shouldn't be perceived as abnormal. As the decades go from the twenties to the eighties, it is joked that sex should progress as follows:

Twenties: tri-daily
Thirties: tri-weekly
Forties: try-weekly
Fifties: try-weakly
Sixties: try-Viagra
Seventies: try-anything
Eighties: try-to-remember

As frequency wanes with age, there are some other noticeable differences. The most rigid erections and most explosive orgasms peak in the teens. These facts have been used to state inaccurately that a male reaches his sexual peak at sixteen or seventeen years old.

This is simply not true. First, many males aren't even sexually active (beyond masturbation) at that age. How could they peak if they haven't even begun to have intercourse? Second, "sexual peak" can mean many different things. Yes, a man's ability to repeatedly reach orgasm is highest while in the teens. If having repeated, quick orgasms were the definition of sexual peak, the claims would be true. However, as sex should be an act of communication and tenderness between two consenting adults, that would be a disappointing peak.

On the contrary, a man peaks sexually when he is able to enjoy a loving, communicative experience with a trusting partner that meets the physical and emotional needs of both parties. That takes practice and experience, and explains why sexual satisfaction is higher among those in monogamous, longstanding relationships than in any other group.

With each increasing decade, erections begin to take longer to rise and ejaculation requires more stimulation. This may actually allow men who had difficulties with rapid ejaculation when younger to experience more relaxed and satisfactory intercourse as they get older. The amount and force of seminal fluid **emission** decreases, as does the intensity of the sensation of orgasm. Understanding the normality of this helps couples adjust so they can enjoy sex in an age-appropriate manner.

SOLO SEX: MASTURBATION

But Onan . . . spilled the semen on the ground . . . and what he did was displeasing in the sight of the Lord, and He slew him also.
—Genesis 38:9–10

When surveys ask how often people have sex, intercourse is assumed to be the meaning. However, sexual expression through masturbation is probably responsible for more total occurrences of sexual activity than intercourse.

Masturbation has been blamed for essentially every ill known to mankind. In earlier days, it was considered evil by most religions. This dates to the biblical reference above involving Onan, whose actions led to his name becoming synonymous with masturbation as the term, *onanism*.

When called upon to impregnate his dead brother's wife so the family genes would live on, he apparently couldn't bring himself to release his seed inside her, knowing the child would be his brother's in the eyes of society. The depiction of God's disapproval left a societal discomfort with *onanism* that persists to this day. (Some experts believe that Onan either experienced **premature ejaculation** or withdrew from the vagina prior to ejaculating, but the term "Onanism" is used solely to describe masturbation.)

Instruments were developed in earlier years to prevent masturbation. To discourage the behavior, gadgets prevented access to the penis in various ways. Some also punished the wearer if any sexual activity occurred, including a spontaneous erection. Some would even push spikes into the penis if erection occurred for any reason. This was sure to cause **performance anxiety**!

Physicians over the years actually blamed impotence on masturbation. Dr. H. Boerhaave proclaimed, "The semen discharged too lavishly occasions a weariness, a weakness . . . foolishness, and impotence."[4] Church youth groups taught of its dangers. The Boy Scout manual warned of the perils.[5]

We now know that masturbation doesn't cause **erectile dysfunction**. In fact, for men who do not have intercourse frequently, masturbation may actually help preserve erections. There is some evidence that "if you don't use it, you'll lose it," so the erections produced during masturbation may actually help preserve normal penile function during these times.

Although we have very little scientific research on the impact of masturbation on penile function, there is reason to believe that filling the **sinusoids** with an erection helps preserve their ability to work. Prolonged periods without filling are believed to increase the likelihood they will atrophy (shrink) and lose their ability to fill and function. If masturbation is the only option to achieve that erection, it may help preserve sinusoidal function until a partner is available to assist.

The only way in which masturbation may contribute to erectile dysfunction is when it is performed too close to attempting intercourse. Due to the refractory period following ejaculation, if men masturbate in the hours (or days when older) before attempting intercourse, they may still be in the refractory period so erections may indeed be impaired. This fact can actually be used to help men with rapid ejaculation. If they masturbate before intercourse, the diminished excitability can sometimes help them hold off rapid ejaculation (see below).

Studies show that virtually all males—and a majority of females— masturbate at some point. This stretches across most demographic groups and ages. Women are surprised to hear that many married men do so. This can be threatening to wives if they suspect this means their husbands have sexual needs not being met at home.[6]

In some ways this is true, but not necessarily in a negative way. Because (on average) men desire sexual activity more frequently than women do, masturbation is an option for them to achieve sexual release that is preferable to infidelity. Even if the sexual needs of both partners are similar, the timing of their desire will often not match.

In addition, masturbation is used by many people simply as a method of releasing sexual or other tension. As long as masturbation doesn't interfere with the relationship, and is not performed excessively or obsessively, the practice is not harmful and probably healthful for anyone whose partner doesn't desire sexual activity at the same frequency.

To answer all the questions about the myths regarding masturbation in one fell swoop, *they are all false.* In the absence of guilt or other mentally negative feelings, there is no physical harm due to masturbation in moderation. Like anything, however, masturbation in excess can lead to problems. This might include irritation of the penis or **urethra**, and can be a sign of psychological obsession or other disorders.

RAPID (PREMATURE) EJACULATION

If insemination were the sole biological function of sex, it could be achieved far more economically in a few seconds of mounting and insertion. Indeed, the least social of mammals mate with scarcely more ceremony.
—Edward O. Wilson, *On Human Nature*, 1978

Rick was a laborer who came to the office each year to be screened for prostate cancer. His father had died of the disease at a young age, so Rick took no chances. The visits were always short, since he always denied any urinary symptoms and said his erections were fine.

When he was approaching fifty, Rick had a different answer to the second question. "I get an erection easily, but I can't keep it up," he said. That sounded more like troubles with **venous insufficiency** (chapter 6), where the blood goes into the penis fine, but flows right back out, causing early **detumescence**. However, on further questioning, it was discovered that he couldn't maintain an erection because he was experiencing rapid ejaculation. He had been able to compensate for this in years past by simply achieving another erection within a few minutes. The second erection was less prone to rapid ejaculation because of desensitization, so with the second erection he and his wife were both satisfied.

Rick's problem was that he had never been able to delay the first ejaculation on any given night through more than a few thrusts. Fortunately, when he was younger his refractory period was short enough that the erection returned before his wife became frustrated. Unfortunately, when his refractory period became longer with maturity, he couldn't regain an erection within a reasonable period of time. Therefore, the complaint of inability to maintain an erection was true, but became a problem only when his increased refractory period kept him from getting a second erection in time. The abnormal issue was the inability to delay ejaculation.

Premature ejaculation is the common term, but since there is no defined normal duration of intercourse prior to ejaculation, the phrase *rapid ejaculation* more accurately describes an ejaculation that occurs before the patient desires. Even the *ejaculation* part of the phrase is inaccurate. Although the obvious outcome is ejaculation (release of semen), it's actually the orgasm that can't be stopped in time.

Even before Onan missed his mark, the condition was recognized in the Greek tale of the conception of mythical King Erichthonius. His father, Hephaestus (the Greek god of fire) attempted to mate with his mother, Gaea. He was excitable enough that despite the fact that "she, being a chaste virgin, would not submit to him," he "dropped his seed on the leg of the goddess." Although the god of fire left disappointed, the story ended happily for the unborn Erichthonius when "she wiped off the seed with wool and threw it on the ground and Erichthonius was produced."

Rapid ejaculation may be *primary* or *secondary*. Primary rapid ejaculation means that the condition has been present throughout a man's sexual lifetime. This is most common. Secondary rapid ejaculation means that a man who previously had good control in delaying ejaculations lost this ability at some point. Rick had primary rapid ejaculation, but had compensated for it until his refractory period became unacceptably long.

Another common presentation of secondary rapid ejaculation involves a man who has always had to concentrate to delay orgasm, but has been able to hold back most of the time so hasn't considered it a problem. However, when he begins having performance anxiety due to mild erectile dysfunction, he may begin to fear he has limited ability to maintain an erection. In order to facilitate or preserve the erection, he may allow himself to become overly stimulated too quickly, leading to the *point of inevitability*. This may cause him to complain of secondary premature ejaculation. Sorting out which came first, the erectile dysfunction or the rapid ejaculation, takes some investigation.

Rapid ejaculation is exceedingly common, as almost every man has at some time had an orgasm more rapidly than he wished. If this is an occasional occurrence, most men will not consider it a problem. However, studies show that somewhere between 22 and 38 percent of men will complain that rapid ejaculation is a regular problem for them.[7]

HOW LONG SHOULD IT TAKE?

Sex is more exciting on the screen and between the pages than between the sheets.

—Andy Warhol

Although Kinsey's data showed 75 percent of men ejaculated within two minutes of penetration, this doesn't fit with what we see in the media. A couple of definitions regarding how long it should take have been made by professional organizations. According to ICD-10, the World Health Organization description of health disorders, ejaculation must occur "within 15 seconds of the beginning of intercourse" to qualify as rapid. Some specialists have tried to define it as an orgasm occurring before the woman has an orgasm at least 50 percent of the time. This is ridiculous, as it assumes that ordinarily women have orgasm 100 percent of the time during vaginal penetration, which is clearly not close to reality. *DSM-IV* is the official diagnostic guideline developed by the American Psychiatric Association. It simply defines premature ejaculation as occurring "before the person [man] wishes." This is probably the best definition available at this time.

In addition, the normal duration of time before ejaculation differs among different populations. Some male-dominated cultures around the world have no expectations beyond an immediate ejaculation. For more egalitarian cultures, men expect to enjoy intimacy longer, and usually feel it is important to satisfy their mates as well. The most common reason men complain of rapid ejaculation in my practice is that they feel they are not meeting the needs of their partners. Indeed, Rick stated that the real reason he sought help was that he felt he was disappointing his wife.

DON'T COMPLAIN

That which distinguishes man from the beast is drinking without being thirsty and making love at all seasons.

—da Ponte, *The Marriage of Figaro*, 1786

Normal in the animal kingdom varies greatly. Most insects ejaculate within seconds. Boar hogs last a matter of seconds, ejaculate up to a liter of semen, and then fall asleep afterwards. Maybe this is the origin of the phrase "men are pigs." Worms stay wrapped around each other for hours, redefining afterplay. Pythons are said to mate for days at a time.

Ejaculation in the animal kingdom sometimes just isn't worth it. Male bees compete for the opportunity to court the queen. One (un)lucky winner gets the right to spend a blissful night in flight with Her Highness, mating in midair. With ejaculation, the penis breaks off and he falls to his death. Whether he actually dies from the breakage or the fall has not yet been determined.

Male black widow spiders face danger every time they score. They must deposit their gift and immediately flee. If their exit is too slow, they confirm the popular name of the species.

Meanwhile, the male preying mantis apparently is inhibited from ejaculating by a reflex from his brain. It is only when his mate bites his head off that he completes the job. That explains the warning not to lose your head over . . .

WHY CAN'T I HOLD BACK?

Younger males usually have had their first sexual experiences alone, when the entire goal is ejaculation. Then, when they begin having intercourse they must change behavior and learn to withhold orgasm—not always an easy switch to make. Most will master the skill within a few tries. Why others fail to develop this ability is unknown, but there is probably a genetic predisposition.

In the past decade, a *neurobiological* explanation has replaced other theories on the cause of rapid ejaculation. It is now believed that, for most men, there is a physical reason they have difficulty delaying ejaculation. Instead of just being "in the head" or due to a learned inability to control orgasm, most men probably have an innate neurobiological reason making them more prone to early release.

Orgasm is essentially a *neuropsychological* event leading to the release of semen. The same event happens in women without emission, obviously, and few women complain of having orgasms too rapidly. The difference seems to be that men detumesce (lose the erection) soon after orgasm, whereas women can continue to have intercourse and may have further orgasms. Life is not fair. If the man could continue to have intercourse after orgasm, it is unlikely there would be any complaint from either partner.

Orgasm occurs when stimulation reaches a point of inevitability. Emission releases semen into the prostate and posterior urethra, yielding the sensation that notifies the man that an orgasm will follow within seconds. Not recognizing this approaching inevitability appears to be part of the problem with rapid ejaculation.

HOLD ON: TREATMENT IS ON THE WAY

He was the trembling excited sort of lover whose crisis soon came and was finished . . . the physical desire he did not satisfy in her; he was always come and finished so quickly.
—D. H. Lawrence, *Lady Chatterley's Lover*, 1932

Until the past couple of decades, it was believed that rapid ejaculation was simply due to a learned inability to stop orgasm. This led to treatments geared to reteach control of the process.

Behavioral modification sounds complex, but may really be as simple as "doing something different." Many men will attempt to distract themselves from the overwhelming stimulation of the moment. This may involve performing mental mathematical calculations, or thinking unpleasant thoughts. Humorist Dave Barry recommends thinking of a female he feels could overwhelm any stimulation.[8] Although he names his own, most men can think of something else to distract them. This approach is less than ideal. Sex is supposed to be a pleasurable experience, so if all the thoughts involved are so negative, enjoyment is sure to suffer.

Attempts at decreasing sensation are another common ploy. Layering several condoms one atop another makes sense, but rarely makes a difference. Masturbation before intercourse makes more sense because of the refractory period (as described previously), but risks thereafter making it too difficult to achieve an erection. If this occurs, performance anxiety may simply add to the problem.

The most common behavioral recommendation is the *stop-start technique*. This is just like it sounds. The patient and partner are instructed to start intercourse but stop all movement or other stimulating behavior when he feels orgasm is imminent. The technique obviously requires the man be motivated to stop the orgasm at the right moment, which sometimes takes more willpower than can be gathered in the heat of the moment. It also requires a patient and supportive partner. Each time the man feels that orgasm is approaching, everyone stops moving to allow the feeling to pass. With practice, he may learn to recognize the sensation and how to suppress it. Sometimes the partner can end up feeling "used" as if in a clinical experiment, so good communication is crucial.

The **squeeze technique** takes advantage of the nervous system's tendency to shut down sensation when overwhelmed. When the man recognizes impending orgasm, he is supposed to withdraw the penis from the vagina and squeeze the glans tightly. This overwhelms the sensations leading to orgasm and delays ejaculation if successful. The biggest problem with this technique is the withdrawal itself. This final stimulation of the penis pulling out of the vagina is often enough to push orgasm beyond inevitability. If so, this ends up being essentially the same act as the withdrawal technique of birth control and can lead to further frustration, as the man ejaculates outside the vagina to the frustration of both parties.

Quiet vagina is essentially a version of the stop-start technique for men who are prone to orgasm immediately upon penetration. The woman gently inserts the penis into the vagina, then sits astride the man without movement or thrusting. This is designed to desensitize him to the stimulating sensations of the vagina. Once mastered, the couple is slowly advanced to the stop-start technique.

RAPID RELIEF WITH MEDICATIONS

When it became clear that Rick's problem described earlier in this chapter was rapid ejaculation, its management was easy to recommend. First, we discussed the nonmedical options described above. He was already familiar with these based on an article he had read in a men's fitness magazine, but they had made no difference.

Without hesitation, he jumped on the suggestion of a prescription for Zoloft. I made it clear that, although it was developed as an antidepressant, the reason it was appropriate for Rick was due to its effect on inhibiting orgasm. Two years later, he doesn't note a change in mood but is able to maintain an erection for ten to twelve minutes most times he has intercourse. His refractory period is unchanged, so on the occasion that ejaculation slips up on him, the evening is finished. However, this only happens every few months, so both Rick and his wife are still satisfied with their current arrangement.

It has long been recognized that certain medications inhibit orgasm. This is most commonly recognized in women, who may complain if a medication makes orgasm difficult or impossible to achieve. However, we can use this finding to help delay ejaculation in men who reach orgasm too easily.

Intuitively, it is a little disconcerting to use a side effect to treat any condition, but this side effect that bothers many women (who are more likely to complain of difficulty with *delayed*, not *rapid* ejaculation) is highly sought after by some men bothered by rapid ejaculation. The reliability of these men returning for prescription refills attests to this approach, as well as the tolerance of any side effects.

Those medications found to delay orgasm are antidepressants. The *tricyclic antidepressant Analafril* seems to have the greatest effect on delaying ejaculation, although it is associated with more side effects than medications in the group called *SSRIs*. The most effective of these appear to be *Paxil (paroxetine)*, *Zoloft (sertraline)*, and *Prozac (fluoxetine)*.

These agents theoretically treat the neurobiological abnormality that makes these men prone to rapid ejaculation by altering the chemical changes that cause ejaculation. Since these medications are antidepressants, they might also cause the changes in the patient that they were originally designed for as well. Namely, they will probably cause some mood elevation. As part of overall health, this effect may be a pleasant surprise to men and to the women who put up with them. The most common side effects include dry mouth, nausea, or dizziness. Rarely, seizures, weakness, or other more serious side effects may be noted.

The dosing of SSRI medications is controversial. Experts disagree over whether a daily dose of these medications is better than simply taking a dose a few hours before intercourse. A daily dose seems to work better in my experience and avoids the sudden realization that intercourse is an option but one forgot to take the medication.

Another medication that helps some men is called SS-cream. This is a new topical cream made from the extracts of nine natural products: *Ginseng radix alba, Angelicae gigantic radix, Cistanchis herba, Zanthoxylli fructus, Asiasari radix, Caryophylli flos, Cinnamoni cortex, Bufonis veneum,* and *Torlidis semen.* The developers didn't explain how they chose the plants they did, but that last one is an intriguing additive.

SS-cream appears to decrease sensation in the **glans penis**, thereby limiting over-stimulation. It is well tolerated, with the only known side effects being some burning or discomfort of the glans in about 20 percent of men who use it. It appears to truly decrease the ease of orgasm, as an overdose actually impairs orgasm in a few men until it wears off. The biggest drawback is that it appears to be another treatment that potentially takes away some of the natural pleasure of sex. Since few men relish the idea of having fewer good feelings during intercourse, this treatment may not catch on.

Finally, Viagra also appears to improve rapid ejaculation, but the reason is unclear. The most likely explanation is that men are more relaxed about their ability to maintain an erection while taking Viagra, so they are more relaxed in general. They don't fear the erection will go away, so they don't have to seek further stimulation in order to maintain the erection.

Obviously, anyone interested in these medications must be under the care of a physician. You should be aware of all effects of these medications prior to taking them, as most of the ones mentioned above were developed for other conditions.

MIND AND BODY

Erectile dysfunction is usually due to physical causes, but because orgasm is a neuropsychological event, therapy for rapid ejaculation should involve the mental aspect. Orgasm isn't "all in your head," but it sure starts there. Many couples will benefit from seeing a mental health professional specializing in sex therapy. This might involve sensate focus as described in chapter 10, but usually involves simply counseling to explore the issues that are causing problems. Choosing the right therapist is obviously key, using the same principles described in chapter 10. Most urologists can recommend someone that deals mainly in sexual health and can make a referral if needed.

A combination of SSRIs and therapy often yields the most satisfying results. This is a situation where one plus one equals more than two. You could guess that most men just want a pill—an easy fix. Therapy requires considerable effort, expense, and can be difficult. Combining medication with therapy can both help the patient and partner through frustrating times and also potentially put a permanent solution in place. Although medications may be needed long-term (and potentially permanently), the combination of counseling and medications often leads to excellent outcomes.

Finally, men experiencing difficulties controlling rapid ejaculation should take a step back to remember why they want to hold off orgasm in the first place. As mentioned, from a biological standpoint a rapid ejaculation does exactly what nature requires—it presents semen to the female partner in an effort to perpetuate the species. However, the real reason men want to hold off ejaculation is that they want to share sexual intimacy with their partner, as well as to please her. Therefore, if ejaculation occurs before both partners are ready and satisfied, it doesn't have to mean that the evening is over. Instead of giving up in disgust, many couples will continue the intimacy even after ejaculation occurs. The altruistic male lover will be willing to provide further stimulation to his mate, even if creativity is required. Recall that few women have an orgasm as a result of vaginal penetration. On the contrary, clitoral stimulation is more likely to cause orgasm in most women, and the penis is actually not the most efficient way for a man to accomplish this. More women can achieve orgasm through oral sex or manual stimulation of the clitoris.

Good communication between partners should allow them to find out what he can do to assure that she is satisfied. Some women don't expect an orgasm to be a routine part of intercourse to begin with. However, if they do, this can be accomplished much more efficiently and reliably with a little romantic creativity as mentioned above. Incorporating foreplay that involves the woman having an orgasm through whatever method she finds most stimulating will assure that these expectations are met. Thereafter, the couple can proceed to vaginal penetration and the pressure (or disappointment) may be off if the man experiences rapid ejaculation.

CONTRACEPTION AND DISEASE PREVENTION

And God said to them, "Be fruitful and multiply, and fill the earth."
—Genesis 1:28

A discussion of normal sexual behavior must include at least a reference in passing to contraception. Sure, sex has been helpful as humans have gone forth to "be fruitful and multiply," but we've done a good job of "filling the earth" as we start the third millennium of the Common Era. As you might suspect, most sex acts these days are recreational, not procreational. Therefore, contraception is part of intercourse during the childbearing years more often than not in our culture.

The primary historical purpose for contraceptive methods was for the prevention of unwanted pregnancy. An additional need recognized more in the past few decades is the prevention of disease transmission. Although we've made strides with the former, the latter is still a problem. Sexually transmitted diseases continue to be a health problem worldwide, and the stakes are rising with the recent emergence of the human immunodeficiency virus (HIV).

Regarding disease prevention, suffice it to say that the adage is true: when you have sex with someone, you are having sex with everyone they ever had sex with, and everyone those people ever had sex with, etc. That doesn't mean sex is a disease waiting to happen—just that precautions must be taken.

The only way to eliminate the risk of sexually transmitted diseases is to eliminate sex. That's not very practical. However, it is practical to use judgment in choosing sex partners you have no reason to suspect are at increased risk of harboring such diseases. In addition, condoms decrease (but don't eliminate) disease transmission. Whether they break, leak, or come off, there is always the chance that sexually transmitted diseases (including HIV) will escape their barrier. Finally, it is well known that certain sex acts, including those that involve trauma to mucosal linings, are more likely to involve transfer of disease. As the man on *Hill Street Blues* said, "Be careful out there."

AN OUNCE OF PREVENTION

> Intercourse even with one's legitimate wife is unlawful and wicked when the conception of the offspring is prevented.
> —Saint Augustine, circa 450 C.E.

Contraception actually means prevention of pregnancy. All contraceptive decisions are personal, involving the desires of the two people having intercourse. However, many religions exert strong influence on contraceptive practices of their followers. Nonetheless, if a decision is made to prevent pregnancy, it is important to understand the likelihood of success with the available measures.

Contraceptive effectiveness is usually judged by the likelihood of pregnancy occurring during a year if a given method is used. The annual pregnancy rate with each method is shown below. Note that many methods of pregnancy prevention are not so reliable. In addition, be aware that condoms are the only contraceptive method that significantly decreases the risk of sexually transmitted diseases. That is, condoms are the only method other than abstinence; but chances are that if you're reading this book, abstinence is not a goal.

Annual Pregnancy Rates Using Available Contraceptive Methods[9]

Implant	2%
Female hormonal injection	4%
Birth control pill	8–9%
Diaphragm	13%
Cervical cap	13%
Condom	15%
Rhythm (periodic monthly abstinence)	22%
Withdrawal (prior to ejaculation)	26%
Spermicidal creams	28%
Female tubal ligation	1–2%
Vasectomy	.01–0.5%

Whichever method of birth control is chosen, it is important to know that sex is never without possible consequence. Enjoy it in health, but be aware of the implications!

KEY POINTS

- The sexual habits of humans are as varied as humans are. Don't worry about what everyone else is doing, but focus on what you and your partner will find to be a satisfactory sex life.
- A healthy sex life should be part of an overall healthy lifestyle for most people. Studies indicate that monogamous people who have active, satisfying sex lives are healthier and live longer.
- Masturbation is a normal and natural form of sexual expression.
- Rapid ejaculation is defined in several different ways, but it does

involve reaching an orgasm more rapidly than members of a couple find satisfying.

- Behavioral and medical treatments for rapid ejaculation have made great strides in the past decade. Most cases can be successfully treated.
- Sex is one of life's greatest pleasures. By the same token, it is one of life's greatest responsibilities. If proper precautions are taken, the chance of disease transmission can be limited, and pregnancy can be achieved on a chosen timetable.

6 Why Me, Lord?
Causes of Erectile Dysfunction

Failure of sexual function is a normal accompaniment of aging....
The attempts to restore potency and libido ... are of doubtful
value. Even if they proved successful, one might still question the
wisdom of putting new wine in old bottles.
— Richard Kern, "The Care of the Aged"

"*Which* one caused my erectile dysfunction?" Edward asked
when he finally got around to admitting the real reason he
came to the office. Like many men, he had made an appointment claiming
the disingenuous diagnosis of "prostate problems." Once the exam room
doors were closed, the truth came out slowly. When men make appointments with the urologist and complain of vague symptoms, they are usually just embarrassed to bring up the real concern. "Prostate problem" often
means "erectile dysfunction," if the right questions are asked.

It was easy to elicit multiple different risk factors Edward had for erectile dysfunction. He smoked and was overweight. A classic hypertensive,
diabetic workaholic well into his sixties, he took propranolol for blood
pressure and alcohol for courage. He and his wife argued frequently—
about their financial status, his snoring, and her weight. "So, which one
caused my erectile dysfunction?" he asked pointedly.

"All of them."

❂   ❂   ❂

Hippocrates believed the rich were at risk of **impotence** because of horseback riding. The rest suffered due to overwork or an unattractive partner. It's hardly ever that simple.

Impotence is typically a *multifactorial* disease. In other words, it is usually due to several different factors in each patient. We must understand all the causes in order to try to control the ones that are responsible in any given person.

THE SMOKING GUN

> A custom loathsome to the eye, hateful to the nose, harmful to the brain, dangerous to the lungs, and in the black stinking fume thereof, nearest resembling the horrible Stygian smoke of the pit that is bottomless.
> —King James I, "A Counter Blaste to Tobacco," 1604

Smoking is the big gun. **Erectile dysfunction** due to smoking is actually a double whammy, limiting blood flow in two ways. Everyone knows smoking hardens arteries. Many people are willing to let this happen to other vital organs like the heart and brain. These vital organs don't get enough oxygen, leading to heart attack, stroke, and other life-threatening diseases. Although the surgeon general warned us decades ago, the threat of these diseases still doesn't stop enough people from smoking.

Erectile dysfunction may not be life-threatening, but smoking is even more likely to kill your sex life. The chemicals in cigarette smoke clog the small blood vessels that are supposed to carry blood into the penis to put pressure into the tire. If these vessels are clogged, there's no way to build up enough pressure for an erection.

The second way smoking limits penile blood flow is by causing spasms while you smoke. This cuts blood flow even more. In addition to the double whammy directly on erections, smoking also hurts erections indirectly by its effect on overall health. If the rest of the body functions less efficiently as a result of an overall deterioration in health, even the world's healthiest penis can't compensate. Finally, if the partner finds cigarette smell or taste objectionable, she will be less likely to be a willing participant. This combination means that if you're reading this book and continue to smoke, you need to stop before doing anything else. Otherwise, your chance of success with any treatment goes down. More importantly, you risk ill health or early death, neither one of which will improve your sex life.

IS SMOKING REALLY BAD?

> Smoking is . . . markedly impolite, an impertinent unsociability.
> Smokers poison the air near and far and suffocate every honest
> person who cannot defend himself by smoking in his turn. Who on
> earth can enter the room of a smoker without getting nauseated?
> And who can stay there and not perish?
> —Johann Wolfgang von Goethe (1749–1832)

The tobacco industry has done a good job of keeping it secret, but the "man's man" depicted in ads smoking a cigarette while riding a horse actually died of impotence, not cancer. If you are asking the question, "is smoking really bad," you have been brainwashed by tobacco company propaganda. Don't listen! Cigarette smoking kills about half a million Americans a year—more than AIDS, automobile accidents, murders, suicides, drug overdoses, and fires combined. Studies estimate the chance of a man reaching normal life expectancy is almost twice as good for a nonsmoker. Quitting early, before too much permanent damage is done, adds almost ten years to a man's life expectancy.[1]

Americans spend over $50 billion each year on smoking-related health costs, on top of the billions spent on the cigarettes themselves. Cigarettes emit too many poisonous chemicals to name, including cyanide, benzene, methanol, acetylene (think blowtorches), carbon monoxide, and ammonia. Another gas emitted is formaldehyde, which is the pathologists' chemical you'll end up bathed in if you don't quit.

Secondhand smoke also affects those around you, especially children. Spouses of smokers are at increased risks of the diseases listed below. Children of smokers have many times more lung problems, including asthma and pneumonia. Sudden infant death syndrome (SIDS) is more likely for babies of smokers. Most importantly, smoking around children teaches them that smoking is acceptable to the people whose approval they most need, so they are likely to carry on this tragic family tradition.

DISEASES WE *KNOW* ARE RELATED TO SMOKING

Erectile dysfunction
Cancer*
Coronary artery disease/heart attack
High blood pressure
Erectile dysfunction
Stroke
Infertility (Not only does smoking harm erections, but also the sperm)
Birth defects
Emphysema (picture old men in wheelchairs with oxygen tubing in their
     noses and catheters in their bladders)
Erectile dysfunction
Bronchitis (remember being awakened in the morning by your grand-
     father's cough?)
Ulcers
Osteoporosis
Rheumatoid arthritis
Erectile dysfunction
Thyroid abnormalities
Incontinence (loss of urine)
Cataracts/blindness
Gum disease/tooth loss (that will help your sex life?)
Did I mention *Erectile dysfunction*?

CAN I QUIT SMOKING?
ONLY IF IT MATTERS TO YOU

If quitting were easy, tobacco executives and many physicians would be out of work. The reason is simple—nicotine is about the most addictive substance known to man. We were taught in medical school that when experimental mice addicted to both nicotine and heroin are forced to choose between the two, they will climb over heroin to get to nicotine. The

---

*Actually, dozens of different types of cancer. We'll regard them as a single disease to keep this list manageable. Just understand that most of these cancers aren't due to damage of the lungs, but rather are due to the effect of smoking on tissues throughout the body. These cancers occur at every stage, from the nose, where smoke enters the body, to the bladder and urethra, where it exits.

tobacco companies have used this addiction for decades to perpetuate the most reliable sales of any product in history. They have even spiked nicotine into cigarettes to make sure no user escapes their grasp. Despite rising prices and punitive taxes, the addicted customers continue to feed their profits almost without question. When the U.S. Postal Service raises the cost of sending a letter to a loved one by two cents, a chorus of disapproval arises, but when cigarettes prices double time and again, few people actually become angry enough to stop buying.

Experts on smoking cessation believe there is no single solution. Some people seem to have a greater potential for addiction, which may be at least partially inherited. Therefore, some people can smoke socially and quit with minimal effort, while those with "addictive personalities" might smoke just a few cigarettes and be addicted for life. These people will have a harder time stopping and will usually need professional assistance. For that matter, anyone attempting any program or drug therapy for smoking cessation should see his physician.

Quitting cold turkey—as a New Year's resolution, for example—is historically the way most people have tried. Unfortunately, only about 4 percent of people will succeed. This led to the marketing success of nicotine replacements. These are available over the counter as gums, patches, nasal sprays, and inhalers. About 10 to 20 percent of people will succeed in the long term using these aids. Hypnosis and acupuncture have been advocated, but proof of their effectiveness is weak.

Bupropion is an antidepressant, marketed under the brand names *Zyban* and *Wellbutrin*, that has helped many people quit smoking. An eight-week course of bupropion increases the effects of *dopamine*, a brain chemical involved in nicotine addiction, plus helps to relieve symptoms of depression while quitting smoking. It is more effective than nicotine replacements and actually *less expensive* than the cigarettes it helps you quit.

The greatest likelihood of success is when a combination of nicotine replacement, bupropion treatment for eight weeks, and counseling is used. Obviously, the person must be motivated as well. Cheating is a sure sign of failure. Sneaking a cigarette within the first two weeks can predict a return to smoking within six months almost 100 percent of the time, so don't even waste time and energy unless you're serious about it.

ARE YOU SERIOUS?

Smoking was a way of life for Ed. He began sneaking cigarettes from his parents and grandparents while still in elementary school. His social structure was unconsciously built around the habit. His friends all smoked, so their evening outings were always spent around a smoky table. Even his relationships at work were with other smokers. The high point of every day was the smoke break in the garage beneath their building. The only people he was close to that didn't smoke were his wife, Debbie, and his two-year-old son, Billy. He had never considered quitting, seeing no reason to, until his father died of a massive heart attack during a church service.

The epiphany came when he was walking up a small hill to the burial site. He began having shortness of breath. Without thinking, he reached into his pocket for a cigarette. Then he began thinking. At thirty-five, he found himself the oldest living person in his family. It was not a good feeling, especially when imagining Billy having a similar experience soon due to Ed's own deteriorating health. The decision was made at that moment to quit. His pocket was quickly emptied and its contents pitched into the nearest receptacle. Debbie was ecstatic.

The first week was tough. He took a few days off work to deal with his father's estate, so his schedule was atypical. He slept poorly and became irritable, but soon found his physical symptoms abating. By the second week he had beaten the addiction.

Things went fine until he returned to work. The first day back, he joined his friends in the parking garage for their usual coffee break. Instead of cigarettes, he brought a cup of coffee to replace his urge for a cigarette. Things went downhill quickly. The smell of smoke provoked a *Pavlovian* response he couldn't withstand. He borrowed one from a coworker and bought a pack from the machine in the break room before lunch.

Disappointed, Ed bought nicotine gum and tried quitting again three days later. He made it through the first coffee break by chewing two pieces at a time, but by lunch, he was borrowing cigarettes again. Now he felt not only addicted, but also a failure for giving up so easily. This only made him smoke more. Debbie was supportive but growing impatient.

Finally, Ed asked for a prescription for bupropion from his primary care doctor. She counseled him on the need to not sneak even a single smoke and recommended smoking cessation classes. He took the prescription and went to let his friends in the garage know how committed he was. Although stressed to the max, he proudly made it through the day.

Friday evening, they joined some friends for drinks at their favorite watering hole. Before they made it to the table, smoke was making its way into his taste buds. When someone pulled out the smokes, Ed reached for one. Debbie grabbed his wrist and pulled him outside. "I thought you were done with this," she cried. It was unclear whether she meant the cigarettes or the lifestyle. Ed's second epiphany ensued.

Smoking is not just an addiction. It's a lifestyle—a ritual. Therefore, you must *denormalize* it to improve the chance of success. This means avoiding situations likely to "make" you smoke. If you go outside the office to the smoking area and hang out with all the other smokers, failure is inevitable. Find a substitute activity unlikely to trigger smoking. Spend that time—and the money you save—sending flowers to your partner. With the improved erections, it will be worth it.

Over that weekend, Ed made the decision to denormalize smoking. At his coffee break, he began hanging out with the nonsmokers inside. He found that he shared many things in common with several of them, but had never had the chance to explore these relationships due to the time he was killing in the parking garage. As these friendships grew, he found that he and Debbie enjoyed the company of many of these people, as well as a completely new group of friends and activities. Their relationship grew, as did his chance of seeing Billy grow up.

ARTERIOSCLEROSIS: HARDENING OF THE ARTERIES MEANS NO HARDENING OF THE VEIN

Any disease that limits blood flow to the penis makes achieving an erection more difficult. Smoking is the most obvious cause of this, but anything that causes hardening of the arteries (**arteriosclerosis**) will do the same thing. Common causes include *hypertension* (high blood pressure), diabetes, excess triglycerides (fats) or cholesterol in the blood stream, or just a hereditary tendency. These all do the same thing by keeping adequate blood pressure from reaching the penis. Notice most of these are interrelated, actually causing each other. High blood pressure causes hardening of the arteries. These hardened arteries can't stretch as well, so cause even further elevated blood pressure. The same goes for high cholesterol and the other conditions listed above. Smoking causes almost all of them.

PELVIC *STEAL*—NOT PELVIC *STEEL*

A specific type of erectile dysfunction due to arteriosclerosis results from **pelvic steal syndrome**. This term may conjure images of stolen parts, but it actually refers to the "theft" of blood away from the penis during pelvic or leg muscle activity required for pelvic thrusting. When the large workhorse muscles of the legs and buttocks spring into action, they send out a demand for increased blood flow so strong that the penis doesn't stand a chance. The blood supply into the area is barely adequate, so most of it is shunted to the muscles and away from the penis.

Men with this phenomenon have adequate blood flow to get an erection. However, there isn't enough reserve to supply the pelvic and leg muscles needed to move that erection around. Therefore, things may start smoothly, but as soon as thrusting begins, blood is diverted to the muscles involved. The thrusts may persist, but the erection doesn't for long. This is sometimes due to *Leriche's syndrome*, which is a generalized poor vascularization of the lower body from hardening of the arteries. The full-blown syndrome is often overlooked because the men usually have so many other serious health problems that impotence is the least of their worries. Therefore we don't fully understand how common this condition is, but it is one of the less commonly reported causes of erectile dysfunction.

NO PENIS IS AN ISLAND: IMPOTENCE AS AN INDICATOR OF MORE SERIOUS DISEASE

The past few years have seen substantial evidence that erectile dysfunction is just part of an overall health deterioration. Arteriosclerosis is a systemic problem that is never limited to just one organ. Just as we know people suffering a heart attack are at risk of other cardiovascular diseases like stroke and hypertension, we know people with penile arteriosclerosis have the same changes going on systemically as well. The high blood pressure, arteriosclerosis, diabetes, and all other systemic diseases stretch all the way to the tip of the penis. That means the penis isn't an island, but it may serve as a poor excuse for a peninsula as well due to diseases affecting the entire body. Therefore impotence isn't just a sexual problem; it's usually an indicator of systemic, potentially life-threatening disease.

Many people with these diseases such as hypertension and arteriosclerosis are perfectly willing to tolerate their risks but then complain to the doctor only when their erections begin to fail. This is often accompanied by an unreasonable perspective on their overall health. They don't see anything wrong with having uncontrolled blood pressure, shortness of breath, and *angina* (chest pain from a heart crying out for oxygen), but they can't imagine why the penis isn't working like new. If their cry for help regarding the penis is noticed by the physician, he can point their whole body, not just the penis, in the right direction.

These coexisting diseases (termed *comorbidities*) also play a role in treatment of erectile dysfunction. Most significantly, the drugs used as first-line impotence therapy can't be used with nitrates (see a complete list of these in chapter 12). If combined, *death is possible*. Moreover, any sudden increased exertion in people with severe cardiovascular problems can lead to a heart attack or stroke, so it is important to know the heart and the rest of the body can handle the effort. Your physician can help you find out.

DIET AND EXERCISE: NO ERECTIONS IF YOU'RE DEAD

Although a knee-jerk answer regarding health is to state that diet and exercise are important, the evidence isn't as clear regarding these factors as it is on smoking. However, the penis will share in the body's overall health (remember, "no penis is an island").

A low-fat diet and moderate exercise have been shown to improve erections. If the body that carries it works better, the penis will perform better. As sex is a physical activity, the body does, or should do, a lot of work during intercourse. If the body can't move efficiently, the penis will be fairly constrained. Shortness of breath looks good when athletic, lithe bodies dance on the sheets of the silver screen. It's not nearly as exciting when sedentary lungs wheeze through a Saturday evening session following a trip to the all-you-can-eat buffet.

Finally, you can't have sex if you're dead. Whatever motivation it takes—sexual, psychological, physical, or otherwise—finding a way to keep in shape is worth it.

VENOUS INSUFFICIENCY: EASY COME, EASY GO

An erection requires trapping of blood inside the **corpora cavernosae** under pressure. If blood runs back out too quickly, the pressure will never get high enough for an erection to occur. Some men suffer from **venous insufficiency**, where the veins allow the incoming blood to run straight through without building up any pressure. The analogy would be pumping air into the tire while it's running out a hole in the other side.

The condition is poorly understood, but venous insufficiency is probably underestimated as a cause of impotence. The diagnosis of venous insufficiency often goes unrecognized as discussed in chapters 7 and 15, but many urologists believe it is responsible for more problems than appreciated. This is probably responsible for many of the failures of the treatments discussed later in this book.

STRESS

Men rarely want to hear this, but stress is a huge risk factor for many diseases. Many physicians believe that stress is at least partially responsible for a majority of all doctor visits. Perhaps first among stress-related diseases is erectile dysfunction. This is because stress attacks erections from both a physical and psychological standpoint. The *psychological* part is obvious, but you'll note in chapter 11 just how important it is. Without understanding and dealing with that aspect, success is difficult to realize.

Physically, stress does two bad things. In the short term, chemicals are released into the bloodstream that cause arterial spasm just like smoking does. In the long term, these chemicals elevate blood pressure and cause irreversible damage to these same blood vessels. In the penis, this leads to erectile dysfunction. Systemically, it risks dysfunction of the heart, brain, and all major organs. If the risk of heart attack or stroke from this doesn't concern you, maybe the risk of erectile dysfunction will inspire you to find a way to stop the cycle. In addition, stress makes us more likely to drink too much, smoke, or find other inappropriate ways to deal with it.

Finally, stress inevitably causes conflict with a sexual partner. This is an example of a **vicious cycle** that should be nipped in the bud. A vicious cycle occurs when one problem causes another, and the second problem in turn causes the first one to get worse. This concept is discussed in detail at several points in the book.

SNORING STOPS SEX:
THE NIGHT'S SECOND-WORST NUISANCE

Snoring is sometimes a symptom of a more serious medical condition known as **obstructive sleep apnea (OSA)**. Both the symptom of snoring and OSA result from a narrowed airway intake during sleep. The body may become starved for oxygen, which obviously isn't good for any tissues, the penis included. Many men with these conditions are impotent.

Why does this contribute to impotence? First, it is commonly associated with obesity (a fat neck is more likely to restrict air flow) and generalized poor health that would also affect sexual function. Second, since these men don't sleep well, they are chronically tired. With only so much energy to give, if they devote most of their energy in bed to breathing, there may not be enough left to devote to sex. In addition, wives of these men often don't sleep well, resulting in their being too tired or irritable to perform. Finally, wives awakened repeatedly by snoring aren't likely to initiate intimacy with their sonorous mates in the middle of the night.

Most of the time weight loss is the mainstay of treatment. When the neck is thinner, the airway may open up adequately to end the problem. However, anyone with severe snoring should be evaluated by his primary care physician or an *otorhinolaryngologist* (ear, nose, and throat specialist).

If the snoring is just a nuisance, there are many options available. Most of these are minimally invasive. *Somnoplasty* is a nonsurgical treatment that uses *radiofrequency coagulation* to stiffen the palate. The procedure uses radiofrequency waves applied to the palate under local anesthesia, usually performed in one to three office visits. These treatments stiffen the palate such that it is less likely to flap noisily as air flows by.

If nonsurgical treatments don't work, surgery to open the airway (*uvulapalatopharyngoplasty*, or *UPPP*) can often be performed under local anesthesia as well. Rare severe cases may require major surgery, but the benefits can be lifesaving. A good resource for sufferers of OSA and snoring is Dr. Derek Lipman's very readable *Snoring from A to ZZZZ: Proven Cures for the Night's Worst Nuisance*.[2] Snoring may not be the night's worst nuisance for everyone, but if it contributes to impotence, it's close.

HORMONAL CAUSES:
THE STORY BEGINS IN THE BRAIN

It was once thought a deficiency of the male hormone **testosterone** was the primary physical cause of impotence. It is now clear that it plays a bigger role with sexual desire than with performance. Other hormonal disorders such as diabetes, thyroid disease, adrenal disease, or pituitary (the master gland) disorders are also associated with impotence.

The complex story of testosterone begins in the brain. The tiny pituitary gland sits at the base of the brain inside the *sella turcica,* a little bony fortress named after the Turkish saddle it resembles. This is perhaps the most protected single site in the human body, designed to safeguard this tiny "master gland" that controls most hormonal processes. The pituitary gland just sits back monitoring the hormone levels under its control. When one becomes low, the pituitary cranks up to stimulate the organ of interest to kick in a little more work.

In this situation, the hormone of interest is testosterone. When the pituitary notices the levels falling, it sends out *luteinizing hormone,* testis fuel designed to crank up testosterone production. When testosterone rises, the pituitary relaxes or finds another hormone that is low to keep it busy.

Sometimes the pituitary-testis team can't keep up due to a failure on either end. The pituitary can become worn out, or a small (usually non-cancerous) tumor can take up too much room in the sella turcica, crowding the master gland so much that it cannot function properly. On the testis end, *primary testicular failure* occurs when the **Leydig cells** just wear out. Thereafter, the pituitary gland can pour out as much luteinizing hormone as it wants and the Leydig cells can't do their part. This would be like pouring more and more fertilizer on your lawn at the end of the growing season. The grass would just continue to do poorly no matter how much stimulation was provided.

Another gland at the base of the brain whose function can affect erections is the *pineal gland.* This tiny gland was of great interest to early anatomists due to its deeply hidden and protected location. To have such an important strategic location, it clearly had to be of importance well beyond its size. French philosopher Descartes declared that the pituitary was actually the seat of the soul—a vital organ if ever there was one.

DIABETES MELLITUS

At least half of all male diabetics become impotent. These men may begin having problems early in life, sometimes even in their teens, especially if they have the more severe, insulin-dependent type (also known as Type I diabetes). Those with Type II, or non–insulin-dependent, diabetes have slower and less severe damage to erections, but a majority of them will eventually develop problems as well.

Diabetic men are at risk of erectile dysfunction for several reasons. First, they have *microvascular disease.* This means they develop damage and narrowing of the smallest vessels, including those supplying the penile tissue. Second, they actually suffer *neurological* damage as a direct result of their underlying disease. This means the nerves to the penis don't send signals as effectively to cause an erection. Frustratingly, the nerves leaving the penis may also decrease the pleasurable signals sent to the brain as well, adding to the difficulty in achieving an erection. That means they are less likely to enjoy penile stimulation, while limiting the stimulatory signals needed to start the erection in the first place. Finally, diabetics may have poorer general health than nondiabetics. As with any other generalized setting of poor health, sexual health will inevitably be part of the equation.

The best thing diabetics can do to try to slow this damage is to keep their glucose levels and blood pressure under control. They obviously can't smoke and have any hope of maintaining normal erections. That doesn't mean diabetics can't have healthy and satisfying sex lives. Rather, they must pay more attention to their sexual health as diligently as they do to their overall health. If they do, success is definitely reachable.

OBESITY: ALL YOU CAN EAT OR ALL YOU CAN HANDLE?

Obesity is linked to impotence for several reasons. First, let's face it, sex is physical. Forty extra pounds makes your jump shot suffer, so why would you be surprised if it cuts performance in bed? Obesity is also linked to hardening of the arteries and decreased oxygen utilization. In addition, as noted above, it causes obstructive sleep apnea. Finally, that extra forty pounds doesn't make your partner more receptive. If she's not interested, you won't be as stimulated.

SURGICAL CAUSES

Any condition that causes damage to nerves serving the penis can cause impotence. This might be due to paralysis from nerve or spinal cord injury, or to neurological conditions like multiple sclerosis. Decreased penile sensation can also accompany any of these conditions. Radiation or pelvic surgery, such as radical prostatectomy, colorectal surgery, or vascular surgery can also damage the nerves involved in erections. Most pelvic surgery, as well as vascular surgery of the lower abdomen, has been associated with erectile dysfunction.

RADICAL PROSTATECTOMY

Almost every man in Dan's family developed prostate cancer by the age of sixty. After his brother was diagnosed with this disease, Dan finally dropped his denial and had his family physician check a PSA blood test to screen for prostate cancer. The PSA was five times the normal level at 20, so his physician referred him for a biopsy through a rectally placed small ultrasound probe. After placing a local anesthetic agent into the area where the nerves enter the prostate, several small (needle-sized) pieces of tissue were obtained and sent to the pathologist.

A few days later, the results confirmed my suspicion. Dan had a high-grade cancer that was fairly bulky and close to the outside of the prostate on physical examination. Although we can preserve the nerves well enough to allow about half of men to retain natural erections after removal of the prostate, I told him I felt there was a high risk that the cancer involved these nerves and that they should be removed to optimize his chance of cure. He was widowed and not sexually active, although he said he got a normal erection through masturbation occasionally. He was much more concerned with survival than sex, so he agreed to have both nerves removed during his operation. He knew that this decision would make it more likely that his cancer would be completely removed and cured, but that the loss of the nerves involved in erections would prevent him from having a normal erection in the future.

The operation went well and Dan resumed most normal activities and function within a few weeks. Although the cancer had indeed grown into the nerves we removed, we were able to get all the way around the tumor with a margin of normal tissue that improved his chance of cure. Things went well for the first two years; he regained bladder control in a matter of weeks and was not bothered by the fact that he couldn't achieve an erection.

During a routine monitoring visit I asked again if he wanted help with erections. Unlike his answer on every previous visit, Dan sheepishly revealed he was seeing someone. They were sexually active, with every-thing except vaginal intercourse. Both partners seemed to care for each other but desired this one remaining pleasure.

Nerve damage from **prostate** surgery used to occur almost 100 percent of the time. The nerves to the penis (called *nervi erigentes* in earlier times) are too small to see with the naked eye. Because surgeons didn't know where they were, these nerves were usually severed during removal of the prostate for cancer, called a **radical prostatectomy (RRP)**. Only after Dr. Patrick Walsh found these microscopic nerves in the early 1980s (see chapter 2) did we know where they were and how to avoid them. Now we can usually protect those nerves during prostate surgery. You may want to check out Dr. Walsh's book, appropriately titled, *Dr. Patrick Walsh's Guide to Surviving Prostate Cancer.*[3]

Unfortunately, these nerves are so small and fragile, they still work only around half the time even if left in place. If they are not cut during the operation, they help improve the chance that the patient will respond to oral medications or other impotence treatments. If we intentionally remove them as we did in Dan's operation, erectile dysfunction is assured.

The other common type of prostate surgery is a **transurethral resec-tion of the prostate (TURP)**. In this operation, a scope is placed through the penis and an enlarged prostate is "cored" or "reamed out" to open a wider channel so men can urinate easier. Since this operation doesn't cut the penile nerves, impotence is uncommon. Still, an occasional man (less than 5 percent) will complain erections are weaker or absent following a TURP. This could be due to nerve injury from the electricity that powers the instrument used to remove tissue, but it may just be due to the psycho-logical idea that prostate surgery can affect erections.

The final issue regarding prostate surgery concerns **orgasm**. Orgasm doesn't require an erection, as noted in chapter 4. This climax is simply a neurological event in which chemicals are released to trigger the feelings that make orgasm so pleasurable. **Emission** is the actual discharge of **semen** into the **urethra**. This is the "point of no return" that is recognized as an inevitable orgasm. It is usually followed quickly by **ejaculation,** which is the actual release of semen out the end of the penis.

To the surprise of most men, emission and ejaculation have nothing to do with the pleasurable feelings of orgasm. Nevertheless, men who undergo prostate surgery should understand they will no longer ejaculate. Since most of these men are beyond their partners' childbearing age, this usually isn't a significant physical issue as long as they understand the difference between emission or ejaculation and orgasm. If they want children, we have a problem. Fatherhood is still an option for many of these men, but they will have to see a specialist in male infertility in order to achieve a pregnancy following most prostate surgery. (At their age, most of them should probably see a psychiatrist as well if they want more children.)

The answer for Dan was **intracorporeal pharmacotherapy** (**ICP**; see chapter 13). Since the only abnormality he had was an interruption of the nerve signals to the penis that tell the blood vessels to open up and fill the tire, it was easy to bypass these signals with an injection that sends a similar signal. An erection could be anticipated within minutes, and both partners were most satisfied with the result.

Radiation treatments for prostate cancer are an alternative to surgery for many men with prostate cancer, and are sometimes given for other pelvic cancer like colon cancer. Radiation also damages the nerves to the penis. Although this damage is much slower in onset than that done by surgery, after three to five years, erectile dysfunction is common in these men as well. Therefore, potency in the short term will be better for men treated with radiation, but down the line they have similar concerns regarding erections and may need similar treatments.

PSYCHOLOGICAL CAUSES

Until very recently, erectile dysfunction was believed to be due to psychological, not physical, causes. The 1970 edition of *Campbell's Urology* stated that impotence is "mostly psychogenic."[4] Based in large part on the Kinsey research on sexual behavior, it was widely held that the problem was "in the mind."

We now know that very few patients are impotent purely for psychological reasons. However, no matter what the original problem is, it's a rare patient that doesn't have a psychological component by the time he considers evaluation and treatment. This can be rooted in classic psychiatric conditions such as depression, anxiety, or psychosis, but is more often due to fear, guilt, stress, performance anxiety, or moral inhibition. The very experience of an inadequate erection automatically adds a psychiatric component. (See chapter 10 for a complete discussion of psychosexual issues.)

Sometimes an underlying psychiatric condition is a major contributor. Mild depression cuts interest and performance, and in its more severe form leads to *anhedonia*. This literally means a total absence of pleasure. If you experience no pleasure in any form, sex is unlikely to happen. Psychoses such as *bipolar disorder* (also known as *manic-depressive disorder*) or *schizophrenia* can be sexually confusing. Sufferers may have decreased sex drive but alternatively may be *hypersexual*, meaning they may exhibit excessive sexual behaviors. Excesses in either direction are unhealthy, and people with these disorders should be in the care of a mental health professional to maximize their chance of success in life as well as in bed. In addition, medications prescribed to treat all psychiatric illnesses can contribute to impotence. Assessing whether the problem is the psychiatric disorder or the medication is sometimes difficult, another reason for aggressive psychiatric oversight.

Finally, psychological "hang-ups" that aren't severe enough to be "disorders" are common (these are as discussed in chapter 10 as well).

RELATIONSHIP CAUSES

Sex is a conversation carried out by other means. If you get on well out of bed, half the problems in bed are solved.
—Peter Ustinov, 1978

A well-known urologist went to the waiting room to let Mr. White's wife know that surgery to implant a **penile prosthesis** had gone well, and that her husband was on the way to the recovery room. He searched futilely around the waiting room for the attractive woman he had met with in the office only days before. Not finding her, he returned to the operating room for his next operation.

During the second case, a call came into the room informing him that the wife was upset that no one had come to speak with her about the operation. She was reassured that things had gone fine, and that the doctor would be out to speak with her as soon as he was finished with the second operation.

When the urologist reentered the waiting room, he still couldn't find the woman that had been so pleased that Mark was to receive an implant. A staff member pointed him instead to a matronly woman in the corner. By the time he got to that side of the room, he realized that the woman he had met during the pre-op visit was not Mrs. White at all. It became quickly apparent that Mr. White had brought his girlfriend to discuss placement of a penile prosthesis, but the real Mrs. White had found out he was having surgery and had showed up to do her wifely duty (one of the wifely duties she apparently still fulfilled).

The ensuing discussion was just the first of many that led to the revelation that Mr. White wasn't quite the simple man he seemed. He came by himself to all future office visits and apparently never had an opportunity to use the prosthesis.

Couples that can't get along in the living room will usually have troubles in the bedroom. In addition, it will take a powerful stimulus to obtain an erection if a man is not attracted to his partner. When a relationship involves bad feelings, the problems don't stop at the bedroom door.

Changes are inevitable as a relationship matures. The emotions of falling in love are powerful, and the early sexual experiences may be powerfully stimulating (as long as the **new partner syndrome** isn't involved—see chapter 10). Later on, the flames that smolder down to embers may not be as arousing.

That doesn't mean sex can't be great as a relationship progresses and develops. On the contrary, most married people state that sex is better in marriage than when single. Better, that is, if both partners put the effort in to make it so. Relationships are like gardens—they only grow if tended. Everyone needs to feel special, so the relationships that thrive usually involve both partners putting in the effort to make each other feel like the most important person in the world.

Unfortunately, many couples take the opposite approach. They may take each other for granted. Even worse, they may bicker and pick each other apart. Neither will lead to grand success in the bedroom.

An extreme example is the man who can't perform with his wife, but has no problem with a girlfriend. This man doesn't need a urologist—he needs a counselor. Or an attorney.

AGING: YOU CAN RUN, BUT YOU CAN'T HIDE

Maturity is a bitter disappointment for which no remedy exists.
Kurt Vonnegut Jr., *Cat's Cradle*, 1963

William and Margaret enjoyed a healthy sex life through the first forty years of marriage. They avoided getting into a rut and met each others' needs essentially every other night. Both were exceptionally healthy and active, playing tennis regularly despite being over seventy. At some point, they both noticed that William had a softer, albeit adequate, erection. It began to take more effort and time. Unless both partners were focused, sometimes he barely got firm enough to penetrate. Margaret was well beyond menopause, so vaginal dryness was not helping.

During a routine office visit, William mentioned the desire to try Viagra. Although it was tempting to write a prescription and move on, I had to ask exactly how much trouble they were having. "It's no problem if I'm well rested, doc," he said. "But if we wait until too late at night, I can barely make it." He noted that a particularly physical tennis game left him with barely the reserves to perform that evening. I inquired about when the last successful intercourse was. "Night before last, so if I can get the Viagra today I should be ready for tonight."

Few couples in their seventies have intercourse every other day, so we discussed their pattern. "We just believe that every other night is right for us, doc. We've always done that, and don't see why we shouldn't continue."

The older men get, the more things can go wrong. All the issues above that contribute to impotence increase with aging. Not only do those conditions become more likely with aging, but also in older men these conditions have had more time to do their slow damage. That doesn't mean sex has to stop with age—just that it may be less frequent and take more effort. However, there is no reason men can't continue to have erections until they are too old to be interested. This can be pretty old.

Because erections take more work—or more time—in older men, often they or their partners get frustrated and become unhappy with the situation. What's the hurry? A more healthy approach is to slow down and enjoy the situation. Foreplay is often the time and situation where couples actually communicate physically, giving more than taking. Enjoying this give and take while waiting for nature to take its course can be most rewarding if neither party gets anxious or frustrated. If both partners are loving and supportive, this may actually allow a sexual relationship to mature to a higher stage.

Many couples unfortunately do the opposite. The men get frustrated, or the women become suspicious or angry. When these feelings emerge, it is crucial to rein them in before permanent damage is done (see chapter 10 for ideas on avoiding these traps). Instead, slow down and enjoy a new phase of life. As the ad says, maybe you're just getting better.

William and I discussed the changes he had noticed in his body, and he conceded that few other physical capabilities were unchanged by this time. His three- or four-hour killer tennis sessions had gradually been pared back to two hours of active, but more leisurely, play. He napped occasionally, and sometimes had barely the energy to do the yard work. He then realized, to his chagrin, that things were just slowing down.

I pointed out that slowing down didn't have to mean stopping. His latency period between erections was now at the point that he really wasn't fully ready two days after the last orgasm. When they discussed this, Margaret confessed that she would like to slow down, but didn't want to disappoint her husband.

A few months later, William boasted that his erections had improved markedly without medications. They had agreed to prioritize quality over quantity, so were making love only about once a week. They did so mainly on weekends, when both were more rested. Margaret had less difficulty with vaginal dryness with the added time between sessions. They increased their foreplay, so both partners were more stimulated by the time penetration was attempted. Life was good again.

PEYRONIE'S DISEASE: BEND BUT DON'T BREAK

> There once was a man from Kent
> Whose tool in the middle was bent
>
> —Anonymous limerick

A *fibrous* (scar-like) plaque develops in the **tunica albuginea** in many men for unknown reasons. This condition is called **Peyronie's disease**. This really isn't a disease, but rather a disorder that is common among men, including Dr. Peyronie. (A dubious honor it is to have your name forever linked to the concept of a bent penis.) These lesions don't stretch during an erection. If just on one side, the other side elongates and creates curvature toward the side of the plaque. Some curvature (thirty degrees or less) is normal, and in fact to be expected. It's no coincidence that the cover of *The Penis Book* has a picture of a banana instead of a cucumber.[5]

It was rumored, but certainly never documented, that the classic curvature of Peyronie's disease played a role in the highest profile case of penile identification. The impeachee reportedly had Peyronie's disease, giving him a bend in the middle that the House Impeachment Committee failed to get a look at.

Because of the **vagina**'s flexibility, this minor curvature doesn't interfere with intercourse. However, patients with Peyronie's disease can have a curvature of ninety degrees or more. This can result in the penis bending at a right angle, making vaginal penetration difficult, if not impossible. If the penis bends more than ninety degrees, it points right back at the owner, making for a dangerous situation!

The worst outcome involves impotence, which happens in a minority of men with the disorder. The plaque itself may not bring patients to the doctor, but the impotence will.

The diagnosis is fairly straightforward even if the penis is not. Nothing else looks or acts like Peyronie's disease, with its curvature and plaques in the tunica albuginea that are easily felt. Many of these patients are concerned about cancer. The good news is that it's not cancer.

The bad news is that, since we really don't understand what it is or what causes it, we also don't know how to treat it. Many remedies have been tried with limited success. Researchers have injected steroids, medications and hormones into the plaques. Radiation and lasers have been tried. However, nothing has really proven effective. When symptoms are minimal, leaving it alone is the best approach. Vitamin E in moderation (400–800 micrograms daily) seems to help, and there are many other reasons to use it, including lowering the risk of cardiovascular disease and cancer. Many physicians prescribe *p-amino benzoic acid*, but this expensive medication has not been proven effective.

At least half of cases get better no matter what you do. The pain, which is present mainly during an erection, usually improves within a year. However, some patients whose curvature continues to worsen may require surgery. Several options exist. Removal of the plaque is theoretically the easiest, but the plaque frequently involves the sensory nerves to the **glans penis**, so decreased sensation is a risk. Despite jokes about genital numbness, no one wants it, so this is best avoided. Another option is sometimes to shorten the opposite side so the penis ends up straight during an erection. The problem with this option is that the shortest side subsequently defines the penile length. As discussed earlier, length is more in the mind of the beholder, but psychologically men bolt at this idea. A final option involves placement of a penile prosthesis, which both straightens the organ out and assures an erection (see chapter 14).

EXTERNAL CAUSES

Many medications have been linked to erectile dysfunction. The usual suspects are medications that treat cardiovascular diseases or hypertension. Unfortunately, it is difficult to know whether the medication or the disease being treated is more at fault. Although reasonable to discuss a change with the prescribing physician, most men's erections don't improve with stopping or changing medications.

The same dilemma occurs with psychoactive medications such as antdepressants, antianxiety medications, and antipsychotic medications. The underlying mental situation requiring the medication may also cause impotence, so stopping the medication sometimes does more harm than good. Depression is the psychiatric condition that is most related to impotence, and recovery from this through therapy and occasionally antidepressants can yield impressive results. Depression causes diminished desire for sex, so correction of the underlying abnormality allows the patient to regain desire. Once desire returns, he can function normally unless any other underlying issues coexist.

The role of medications in erectile dysfunction is complex. Although it sometimes seems impotence began around the time a new medication was prescribed, it's easy to overlook the fact that new medication was started to treat some disease or problem. The pill to treat your *angina* (chest pain from heart damage) might cause impotence, but it's more likely the arteriosclerosis and heart disease that required the prescription that are the real culprits. Likewise, the antidepressant may cause problems, but the depression might be keeping the penis down as well.

MEDICATIONS BELIEVED TO CONTRIBUTE TO ERECTILE DYSFUNCTION

This list of medications reported to cause impotence is not exhaustive, but most of the frequently mentioned ones are below. Notice that many of them are cardiovascular medications or antidepressants. Although many more medications have been reported to contribute to erectile dysfunction, the most common ones are included.

Accupril
Aldactone

Aldactazide
Aldomet (Methyldopa)
Altace
Amytriptyline (Elavil)
Catapres (Clonidine)
Capoten
Cimetidine (Tagamet)
Corgard
Digitalis (Digoxin)
Dilantin (Phenytoin)
Hydrochlorothiazide (Dyazide, Maxide)
Inderal
Ketoconazole (Nizoral)
Lotensin
Lopressor
Maxzide
Minipress (Prazocin)
Moduretic
Monopril
Niacin
Normodyne
Phenobarbital (and all barbiturates)
Prozac
Sectral
Tenormin
Toprol
Zestril
Zoloft (Sertraline)

RECREATIONAL DRUGS AND ALCOHOL

> Lechery, sir . . . it provokes the desire but takes away performance.
> —Shakespeare, *Macbeth*, act 2, scene 3

Many recreational drugs other than tobacco affect erections. Alcohol is number two. Many men increase alcohol intake when experiencing erectile dysfunction. There are two reasons for this. Seeking a little manhood in the bottom of a bottle is the first—a time-honored idea that has never worked.

The porter in *Macbeth* understood the role of alcohol; although the alcohol makes you aroused, bolder and braver, it actually depresses the central nervous system. That means that, instead of stimulating, it actually blocks the ability to perform sexually. Men under the influence begin to think of themselves as Don Juan but actually may end up performing like Don Carlos.*

The second effect of alcohol on erections is longer term. Permanent harm results from prolonged intake of alcohol, including *cirrhosis* (liver damage), malnutrition, brain damage, and depression. These may contribute (especially cirrhosis) to testicular dysfunction and shrinkage, obviously not good for erections. Instead of seeking sensuality in a bottle, men usually need to face their anxieties or inadequacies in a more direct manner.

Marijuana can lower testosterone levels and sperm count. Steroids used for bodybuilding do the same thing and can cause irreversible shrinkage of the testicles. In addition to all the other serious health issues than can occur, those abs of steel won't be enough to overcome the negative effect on your love life.

BICYCLING: SOMETHING GOOD OR BAD BETWEEN YOUR LEGS?

> Riding should be banned and outlawed. It's the most irrational
> form of exercise I could ever bring to discussion.
> —Irwin Goldstein, M.D.

The nineties brought a surge in bicycling among men. Big bucks were spent on the newest carbon-fiber or titanium-frame bicycles in order to get in shape and look cool on the newest technology. Researchers, primarily led by Dr. Ira Goldstein of Boston, rained on their two-wheeled parade when numerous reports arose of erectile dysfunction among these otherwise healthy specimens.

These men were doing everything right—exercising, keeping their weight down, eating right, and preserving their mental health. Unfortunately, it is likely some of them also sat on the *internal* **pudendal artery**, the crucial inflow of blood for erections, so much that they obstructed it. The injury kept blood flow from reaching the penis. The warning signs were there, including penile numbness or **paraesthesias** (weird sensations) after long rides.

---

*The leader of the Spanish Hapsburgs, the family whose reign ended due to the impotence described in chapter 2.

The evidence that the pressure of the bicycle seat was the culprit "mounted" until it became clear that excessive bicycling is a risk factor for impotence. Defining what is excessive is difficult of course, but common sense has to play a significant role.

The catch-22 is that men need the cardiovascular workout and weight loss that bicycling affords in order to minimize impotence. Thinner men have less padding to protect the pudendal artery from the bicycle seat, but heavier men put more pressure onto the artery because of the added load. Damned either way.

Getting weight off the seat on a regular basis helps. Doing so for even a few seconds helps allow the compressed tissues to refill with blood. One option to avoid perineal pressure completely is a recumbent bicycle, but most men are still too concerned about looking "dorky" in these, so they haven't caught on yet.

A cottage industry immediately arose to build bicycle seats whose manufacturers claimed would eliminate this problem. Despite the marketing, there is no proof yet these seat pads work. However, it is probably worth considering if you ride on a regular basis. Tilting the front of the seat downward also minimizes pressure applied to the wrong place as well.

We haven't heard the end of this controversy. The best recommendation at this point would be to get plenty of aerobic exercise. If this exercise includes bicycling, avoid prolonged pressure on your perineum. *Get up out of the seat every few minutes.* Although, as noted, the effectiveness of seats specifically designed to prevent impotence has yet to be proven, it can't hurt to look carefully at these before making your own decision.

If permanent arterial damage occurs to bicyclists, surgery to bypass the arteries may be the only option. (This is discussed in chapter 15.)

Amazingly, fifteen hundred years ago Hippocrates theorized excessive horseback riding caused impotence among the moneyed citizens of Scythia based on trauma to the perineum. It is unknown whether the saddle manufacturers at the time tried any innovations.

PENILE FRACTURE: COITUS INTERRUPTUS WITH A "POP"

Occasionally during intercourse, he zigs when she zags, resulting in *penile fracture*. This is an easy diagnosis. Following an audible "pop," the penis goes immediately soft (you're surprised?), turns black and blue, and makes the owner most unhappy. This is truly a fracture or tear of the tunica albuginea. Surgery to repair this tear must be performed quickly in order to minimize the chance of permanent impotence.* If treated early, penile fracture may not cause permanent damage. It's the one risk factor least likely to go unnoticed or unreported.

PRIAPISM: TOO MUCH OF A GOOD THING

> They [patients with priapism] are not at all relieved [of the erect member] by . . . repeated acts of sexual intercourse. . . . For the most part the patients die on the seventh day.
>
> Arataeus the Cappadocian, first century C.E.

Despite the impression Hollywood gives, an erection should never last more than four hours. If it does, the penis receives inadequate oxygenation and damage begins to occur. This is called **priapism**, named after the Greek god Priapus, and is a most unpleasant situation. The penis is painful. Intercourse is the last thing on the mind of the victim.

Many cases in the past were due to sickle cell disease or some medications. Most cases at this point are due to injection of medications into the penis used to cause an erection as discussed in chapter 13. Less common causes include trauma, blood clots, neurological conditions, malignancy, or infections.

If it is due to penile injections, treatment might be as simple as aspirating out the blood and medication by using a needle. If this doesn't correct the situation, a medication can also be injected into the penis that will block the increased blood flow that is causing the problem.

More difficult cases require an urgent trip to the operating room. Although sometimes the erection goes away with induction of anesthesia, some type of operation is usually required to shunt blood out of the penis. An unfortunate number of men suffer permanent erectile dysfunction even with ideally performed, expedient surgery. Those who delay too long are almost assured of it.

---

*Discretion should be taken in whom you let sign the cast.

ADDITIVE RISK: PUTTING IT ALL TOGETHER

Most men have enough reserve that a single one of these insults won't be enough to cause erectile dysfunction. However, when they start to add up, treatment may be needed. There is almost always a combination of physical and psychological factors in play. The psychological response to the physical problem is usually the final blow.

Does this mean it's too complex, so you should give up? Of course not. Unfortunately, most patients want a simple one-word answer. Nevertheless, when we go over the above list most people can recognize the *multifactorial* nature of their condition and are willing to consider this when deciding on treatment options. Some of their risk factors (smoking, obesity, medications) can be changed, but many others can't. We can't make you younger. Diabetes and hypertension have not been cured, but they can usually be controlled with some combination of medication and lifestyle change. Overindulgence of alcohol, illicit drugs, or food can be corrected. Although difficult, smoking can be stopped if it's important to you. If the risk of early death doesn't motivate you, the early death of your sex life may.

SO WHICH ONE CAUSED
MY ERECTILE DYSFUNCTION?

At the beginning of this chapter, Edward wanted to know the one reason he was impotent. Obviously, most of the things noted earlier probably played a role. However, knowing what caused it doesn't automatically solve the problem. Many of his risk factors were irreversible. He could do nothing about his age except add one to it each year. He could treat his hypertension and Type II diabetes, but the medications had erectile dysfunction as possible side effects. The long hours he worked didn't bring in enough money to prevent its short supply from being a source of stress in the couple.

Nevertheless, he could make some changes. The propranolol for his blood pressure was switched to another pill that didn't affect erections as much. With an exercise and dietary program, he was finally able to get off medications altogether. He stopped smoking, and drank alcohol responsibly and only for pleasure. With the weight loss, the snoring became less problematic. Both he and his wife slept better.

Finally, the positive changes in Edward allowed him to approach his wife in a more constructive manner as well. They began discussing issues reasonably instead of arguing. She began her own dietary and exercise program. They began to find each other more attractive, which in turn caused each to be more motivated.

After taking Viagra for several months, Edward cancelled an appointment without rescheduling. At a later social event he leaned over and told me that he no longer needed the help. His health, and that of his marriage, had before then been deteriorating on multiple levels without him putting up any resistance. It was only when his sex life was on life support that he made the changes. His penis may have saved his life.

KEY POINTS

- Almost all cases of erectile dysfunction are due to several different causes working together.
- If the "straw that broke the camel's back" is one of the reversible causes such as smoking or anxiety, this can be targeted as a way to restore erections permanently.
- Some causes of erectile dysfunction are irreversible. Fortunately, effective treatments are available to overcome them if this is the case.
- If smoking doesn't kill you first, it will probably kill your sex life at some point.

7

Diagnosing Impotence
It's Not Hard

I know it when I see it.
—Potter Stewart, U.S. Supreme Court Justice

*I*mpotence was a cause for annulment of marriage in sixteenth- and seventeenth-century France. Tens of thousands of cases appeared before the courts, necessitating establishment of a five-stage standardization of the diagnosis. The husband's confession and a neighborhood inquiry were the relatively nonstressful first two stages. A three-year trial period followed.

Then things got serious. The fourth stage involved cross-examination by judges and a genitourinary examination of the husband and wife by the local surgeon (who also happened to be the local barber). The "test of congress" was the final stage: the husband and wife were brought before a public gathering of doctors, surgeons, matrons, and judges in order to allow a man to try to prove his potency. If he was up to the task, annulment was refused. If for any reason (including the inevitable performance anxiety) his erection failed to show up in court, the marriage was over.[1]

You don't need a medical degree to diagnose **erectile dysfunction**. All you have to do is listen and look. If a man says he's impotent, who can argue? For that matter, if his partner says he's impotent, she's clearly the expert opinion of the moment. Therefore, the very complaint of erectile dysfunction is enough to establish the diagnosis.

127

The American Urological Association and the 1992 National Institutes of Health (NIH) Consensus Statement defined it as "the inability to achieve or maintain an erection sufficient for satisfactory sexual performance." Notice that quantification or other confirmation is not included in that definition

The *First International Consultation on Erectile Dysfunction* convened in Paris in 1999 to review all the scientific information available on erectile dysfunction in the ambitious hope of reaching a consensus on management. Cosponsored by the World Health Organization (WHO) and *Société International d'Urologie*, they defined erectile dysfunction as "the consistent or recurrent inability to attain and/or maintain penile erection sufficient for sexual performance." They required at least a three-month duration of problems (thereby qualifying as "consistent") unless there was a clear cause such as trauma or surgery. They stipulated that the term *erectile dysfunction* excluded penile curvature, **priapism**, painful erection, **rapid ejaculation**, desire abnormalities, or orgasmic abnormalities.

The most important distinction in diagnosing erectile dysfunction is determining whether it is *primary* or *secondary*. Primary impotence indicates that the man has *never* had the ability to achieve satisfactory erections. This is exceedingly rare and should be investigated both physically and psychologically due to its exceptionality. Most cases involve secondary erectile dysfunction, where the man has previously had normal erections, but at some point loses his ability to perform.

Much is written on validating the diagnosis, but no matter what, it works or it doesn't. Most urologists therefore define it as Justice Potter Stewart defined pornography: we know it when we see it. Basically, if the male says his erection is inadequate to meet the demands of he or his mate, he is impotent no matter how you define it or what the tests show.

"IMPOTENCE" OR "ERECTILE DYSFUNCTION": WHO CARES?

> The medicalization of sexuality may thus be either a threat or a blessing.
> —Roy Porter, *The Greatest Benefit to Mankind: A Medical History of Humanity*, 1997

The term *impotent* literally means "without power." This might explain why the disorder seems to be nonexistent in the White House. This term has been criticized as being too negative, as it implies that erections and power are synonymous.

Therefore the older term is politically incorrect to some. Thus the more conciliatory term *erectile dysfunction* came into vogue in the past couple of decades. This phrase really took off with the marketing campaign waged by Pfizer for their launch of Viagra. Since it was acceptable for a former senator to speak of his own erectile dysfunction, it must be acceptable for everyday conversation. For a while, the "ED" phrasing was common, but enthusiasm for that term seems to have faded in the lexicon. Whatever you call it, if a male can't get it up, he has "the problem."

The term *erectile dysfunction* may mean more than the obvious. Technically, *dysfunction* means "bad function," so any problem with erections could be considered erectile dysfunction. Despite exclusion of these terms by the International Consultation (the Paris consensus conference), that might mean rapid (premature) ejaculation, penile curvature (**Peyronie's disease**) or any difficulties a man has involving an erection. Since the International Consultation was a consensus conference and not a binding or official organization, their definition isn't the last word.

Finally, the term **impotence** is still used occasionally as well. Though it is used by the general public, it is not commonly used in the urology office any more.

THE GOAL-ORIENTED APPROACH TO MANAGEMENT

The reason we don't feel that diagnostic testing is required for most cases is based on the concept of goal-oriented treatment. That means we will treat the problem in order to overcome it using the same options in most cases without regard to its cause. Therefore, when the option chosen restores reliable erections, it usually doesn't matter why. Don't argue with success. For the same reason, if it doesn't restore reliable erections, we must resort to another treatment no matter what. Testing usually doesn't change that. The only significant exception to this is when impotence is primarily psychogenic. Addressing the psychological issues may put an end to the problem so pursuing this is often worth the effort.

With few exceptions, most patients will be best served by the **goal-oriented approach**, which is also discussed in chapter 16. However, for those who need a more definitive diagnosis, see below.

WHEN IS IT APPROPRIATE
TO DO MORE INVOLVED TESTING?

Most men will respond appropriately to the goal-oriented approach and should be offered treatment options with little or no diagnostic tests. However, some men want more specifics. If needed to satisfy either the inquiring mind or the insurance company wanting documentation, some tests can provide an exact diagnosis.

There are three main reasons for people to go beyond the goal-oriented approach and pursue more intensive testing. The most common is the man, typically young and healthy, who has erectile dysfunction and can't understand why without any identifiable risk factors. Sometimes these men "just have to know the reason." Without the information, these men may not be able to accept their situation in order to move on to management. The tests may show low blood flow or some other abnormality to explain why an otherwise healthy man is having erectile dysfunction. More likely, investigation will show that things are normal anatomically, which implies psychological issues are the cause. This knowledge can be helpful, since it allows them to address the underlying problems instead of looking for "something wrong."

The second reason further testing may be needed is when the physician suspects something unusual. Most commonly, this is when a man doesn't respond as expected to treatments. For example, if a man fails to regain erections using oral medications and injection therapy, he may have more troubles than meet the eye. A venous leak or vascular abnormality (see chapter 15) might explain the failure to respond. Another reason to believe things may be complex may relate to a history suggestive of injury to the blood supply to the penis. A remote history of pelvic trauma or a significant bicycling history might make the physician suspect arterial injury. Tests to determine if this is the case might be in order.

The final reason an investigation is performed is for research purposes. Although we know a lot more about erectile dysfunction now than we did two or three decades ago, there are still many things we don't fully understand. Continuing this research is the only way we will ever get closer to eliminating erectile dysfunction altogether. Though we may never eradicate it completely, we have the chance through quality research to decrease its incidence greatly, and the chance to treat those whose disease we can't prevent.

The International Consultation designated several levels of recommended investigation depending on the clinical situation, dividing them into *recommended, optional,* and *specialized.* They concluded that erectile dysfunction should usually be considered a confirmed diagnosis based primarily on the patient's description of the problem. Therefore they *highly recommended* a comprehensive sexual, medical, and psychosocial history (doctor interview) be obtained in addition to a focused physical (genital) examination in all patients. In addition, they recommended that a standardized scale be used to assess the severity of the erectile dysfunction by a questionnaire.

If further investigation was needed, they less strongly *recommended* testing through *fasting glucose* or *glycosylated hemoglobin* (to check for diabetes), *lipid profile,* and hormonal studies to assess the elements involved in male hormones. They concluded that more involved investigations including psychological evaluation and more involved laboratory testing is *optional* and reserved for cases that are more difficult. Finally, they stated that uncommonly, an in-depth psychological evaluation could be obtained, and that assessment of erection quality should be performed only in rare, complex cases where surgery was being considered (see chapter 15).

TALKING TO THE PHYSICIAN: MEDICAL HISTORY

Dialogue between the physician and patient is the cornerstone of erectile dysfunction management. Although some of the questions a physician will ask are included on the self-administered questionnaires described below, there is no substitute for a heart-to-heart discussion between the patient and his physician.

Ideally, his partner will be part of the conversation, but in the real world that is uncommon unless problems escalate or don't respond to early intervention. On the initial visit, most men come alone, and often aren't keen on leading the conversation. Hopefully, your physician will take the initiative and press for a further exploration of the problem. Physicians are human too, so, unfortunately, not all of us are comfortable discussing sexual issues. The vast preponderance of urologists, nevertheless, are comfortable with the topic, so they will usually be open to pursuing the issues.

The questions that should be considered by both patient and physician revolve around finding out how severe the erectile dysfunction is and whether it is reversible. The most important questions follow:

1. *How long have you been having trouble?* This implies things have gotten severe. Often, the longer it takes to develop a condition, the longer it takes to recover.
2. *When was the last time you successfully completed intercourse?* If it has been a long time (several months or longer), correction will be probably require more effort than if you have achieved success more recently.
3. *Did the problem arise suddenly or gradually?* A sudden onset indicates a significant or complete psychogenic component.
4. *Do y*ou ever *have a normal erection, including upon awakening in the morning*? An affirmative response indicates a psychological component.
5. *What is your partner's response to the problem?* For one thing, sometimes the problem is a concern to the man, but the woman may not be interested anyway. In this situation, the man may mistakenly believe he is disappointing his partner, but she may not care. If this is the case, the man needs to make sure he clarifies whether he really wants to treat the problem. If both parties are disinterested in sex, they may be better off facing this fact and choosing to pursue it no longer. If the opposite is true and the partner desires sexual activity beyond what he is currently capable of providing, then his altruism is justified and every effort should be made to assure he can keep up his end of the bargain.
6. *Is there a significant bend or pain in your penis?* Although a minor curvature is expected in all penises, a curve that impairs penetration or pain with erection suggests Peyronie's disease (discussed in chapter 6).
7. *Are there any psychological issues you think are playing a role?* This is often the most revealing question and may open the door for patients to say what's on their mind. If the patient has suspicions on what the problem with his erection is, he is often right.

PSYCHOSEXUAL HISTORY

Peter was a music professor at a local college who readily admitted that the reason he was seeking assistance for erectile dysfunction was that his wife insisted on it. He denied interest in having intercourse, and stated that their primarily platonic relationship was all that he expected or wanted. For that matter, Caroline wasn't especially motivated to have intercourse. Rather, she felt it odd that he never initiated intimate contact, although he usually performed adequately until the last few months. She thought this seemed odd and must indicate some health problem.

He was a handsome, well-dressed man of forty-eight that physically seemed to match her own stately beauty. Their marriage was sound, if unspectacular, with two sons in their early twenties. Our initial visit didn't reveal any obvious medical issues, and his physical examination was normal. A testosterone level obtained by his referring physician indicated a normal hormone level.

It seemed that there was more than met the eye in Peter and Caroline's situation. Asked about childhood issues or unresolved sexual concerns, he just said his work was his passion, and that sex wasn't a priority. "There is no other woman," he denied when specifically asked.

That was the clue. I followed up with "Have you suspected homosexual tendencies?" That hit the nail on the head.

Sometimes the conversation should involve more than a cursory discussion of these issues. Unresolved psychosexual issues from childhood hang on longer than most people want to believe. Occurrences from earlier in life lay the groundwork for future sexual interactions. Sometimes this involved sexual conflict based on the parents' contentious relationship. More distressing is trauma left over from sexual abuse earlier in life. These issues may be suppressed and resurface during sexual situations years later.

As the son of a religiously conservative family, Peter had suppressed his homosexual feelings since adolescence. He had never acknowledged his orientation publicly until that moment. Once the topic was opened, he conceded that he had always known he found men attractive, although he had never acted on his inclinations due to his upbringing and his social standing. Although Caroline was a striking woman, his attraction to her was as his best friend, not a lover.

The complexity of Peter and Caroline's issues clearly required psychological, not urological intervention. He arranged a much-needed session with a therapist.

PHYSICAL EXAMINATION

Although treatment is often based purely on the patient's report of erectile dysfunction, all patients should be examined at least cursorily in order to assure there is no obvious physical cause. Certain genetic conditions associated with erectile dysfunction are suspected by a distinctive body shape. For the patient receiving good medical care otherwise, this will be focused mainly on the genitourinary organs.

The penis is checked for lesions and Peyronie's disease as noted earlier. The testicles are examined to assure that their size is normal. If they are small, hormonal deficiency is suspected. Enlargement of a testis is usually just from fluid around it, called a *hydrocele*. If the patient appears to have an extra testicle, it is usually that we're seeing just a fluid collection called a *spermatocele*.

A prostate and rectal examination are usually performed only in older men or when there is suspicion of a more complex problem (see below, "Neurological Testing"). A rapid assessment of an intact pelvic innervation can be performed using the **bulbocavernosus reflex.** This reflex is performed with an examining finger inside the rectum. When the penile tip is stimulated, most commonly with a quick squeeze, the *anal sphincter* muscle should contract around the examining finger if the neurological reflexes are intact. If it doesn't, a neurological problem is suspected of playing a role in the problem.

Some patients will exhibit erectile dysfunction as the initial reason they see a physician. As noted in chapter 6, impotence is often just a penile manifestation of a systemic disease like **arteriosclerosis**, *hypertension (high blood pressure)*, or diabetes. Therefore, unless these conditions have been eliminated in any given patient, the physical examination should include a measurement of blood pressure, a quick listen to the heart and key arteries, and a check for diabetes.

A more involved discussion of a physical examination and a visit to the urologist's office is found in chapter 9.

LABORATORY TESTING

The International Consultation recommended laboratory testing be individualized. Most patients will have a blood test to assess **testosterone** levels. If this hormone is low, replacement can help libido and might help erections as well. A low testosterone level can be an indicator of more serious disease, including a benign brain tumor, so further investigation is appropriate. In addition, if hormonal abnormalities are suspected, further blood tests are performed to assure that there is no more serious cause.

Diabetes is an abnormality of insulin metabolism that can sometimes be silent with no obvious symptoms. Erectile dysfunction is sometimes the first reason the patient goes to a physician and finds out he has diabetes. Therefore, a urinalysis is performed to check for sugar in the urine. If sugar is found in the urine, a blood test is done to confirm the diagnosis, and the patient is referred to someone appropriate to manage the problem.

Measurements of cholesterol and triglycerides (fats in the bloodstream) are taken only in patients suspected of having systemic cardiovascular disease or in those with family histories suggesting they have a high risk. Liver function tests, chemistry profiles, blood counts, and other specialized tests are infrequently needed unless the patient's general health indicates the possibility of any other medical problem that might contribute to erectile dysfunction (see chapter 6).

SEX SCORES: QUESTIONNAIRES

Multiple different sexual function profiles and erectile dysfunction questionnaires are available. The all end up having initials like BMSFI (Brief Male Sexual Function Inventory), EDITS (Erectile Dysfunction Inventory for Treatment Satisfaction), or **IIEF (International Index of Erectile Function)**. The IIEF has enjoyed the most popularity and is currently the standard required for most medical publications reporting research regarding erectile dysfunction. The IIEF started out as a fifteen-question list, but its little brother, the IIEF-5, cuts right to the bone with five questions:

1. How do you rate your *confidence* that you can get and maintain an erection?
2. With sexual stimulation, *how often* have your erections been sufficient to allow for penetration (entering your partner).
3. During sexual intercourse, *how often* were you able to maintain an erection after penetration?
4. During sexual intercourse *how difficult* has it been to maintain your erections until completion of intercourse?
5. When you attempted sexual intercourse, *how often* was it satisfactory to you?

The IIEF-5 uses a scale to quantify the answers to the above questions:

0. I'm not at all sexually active or I haven't tried intercourse.
1. Very low or almost never/never.
2. Low, rarely, or very difficult.
3. Moderate or occasionally.
4. High or most of the time.
5. Very high or almost always.

The IIEF is the most common sexual inventory scale in current use, and has been validated in at least seven languages. The language of love is truly international.

A very user-friendly sexual inventory scale is the Sexual Health Inventory for Men (SHIM). Developed at Pfizer as a close match to the IIEF-5, this five-question query gives a sexual dysfunction score in minutes that allows a man to quantify how much of a problem he is having. It is available on the Pfizer Web site at www.viagra.com/consumer/about Ed/findOutShim.asp. Although a specific number isn't "abnormal," a poor score helps some men feel more justified in seeking help. A number below 21 implies "signs of erectile dysfunction" and encourages the test taker to seek medical advice. A link on the score page allows you to print out your responses and score in order to facilitate initiation of the discussion with a physician.

PHYSICAL OR PSYCHOGENIC?

The biggest question in most cases of erectile dysfunction is whether the problem is mental or physical. As discussed in chapters 6 and 10, there is usually a combination of both. However, if we know that it's primarily mental, that might direct treatment toward a more permanent solution, so it is helpful to attempt to find that out.

The most important feature in differentiating between mental and physical causes involves the manner in which onset of impotence was noted. Physical causes usually are gradual in onset and their severity tends to be constant and unrelated to circumstances. In contrast, psychogenic impotence tends to be situational and often occurs without warning. A new partner (see chapter 10) may trigger anxieties that lead to sudden failure in a man who has had no problems in previous relationships. Another common scenario is in the man who notices slight difficulty in maintaining an erection. He often will experience a sudden increase in anxiety as he fears that he may not succeed the next time he tries to have intercourse. This very fear can be crippling.

As mentioned, physical causes usually will end up leading to mental exacerbation as well. However, the mental angst usually follows a period when a man or his partner begins noticing a gradual decline in quality and rigidity of the erection. The mental part just becomes the coup de grâce.

Unfortunately, there is no diagnostic test to confirm psychogenic impotence. Therefore, if a definitive differentiation between physical and mental is necessary, the next step may involve testing to assure that the man is physically capable of achieving an erection.

The easiest way to know if he is physically capable is to note whether the penis ever becomes erect. Some men unable to achieve or maintain an erection with a partner will have no problem with masturbation. We must be specific on this question, however, as an erection is not *required* for **orgasm**. That means that some men with total erectile dysfunction will have an orgasm with masturbation without achieving any **tumescence**. That is in contrast to the man who has a full erection with masturbation and then achieves orgasm. In the latter instance, erectile dysfunction is undoubtedly primarily psychogenic and should be addressed as such.

NOCTURNAL ERECTIONS: THE SUN ALSO RISES

> It doesn't make any difference to a woman.
> —Georgette, to the impotent protagonist Jake,
> in Ernest Hemingway's 1926 novel, *The Sun Also Rises*

A more likely way to show that a man can achieve an erection is by confirmation of penile erections during *rapid eye movement* (*REM*) sleep. REM sleep is the deepest phase of sleep, and is associated with spontaneous erections unrelated to sexual stimuli. This occurs mainly during the latest part of the sleep cycle, so it is more likely to cause *nocturnal* (nighttime) erections as the sun also rises.

If present, it implies normal plumbing, hormones, and electrical connections, so a mental cause may be suspected for the erectile dysfunction. Caution must be applied, however, as the presence of nocturnal erections doesn't rule out physical causes. It just makes them less likely to be the only problem.

A final note on nocturnal erections: men often incorrectly think these erections are due to a full bladder. This observation comes from the fact that they awake needing to void, so the erection springing from their REM sleep is sitting there in their hands as they empty the bladder. By the time the bladder is empty, the penis usually is as well, leading to the errant correlation.

Some men will even use this observation in an attempt to self-treat. They conclude that if they attempt intercourse after filling the bladder with a few beers, the penis will gain the girth needed. These elements are unrelated, so this home remedy is bound for failure. In addition, the beers used for bladder filling usually only complicate things if consumed in excess, as discussed in chapter 6.

Nocturnal emission is often mentioned along with nocturnal erections. This is an unconscious **ejaculation** during sleep that is unrelated to sexual stimulation. Although it sometimes occurs during an erotic dream, it can also be asexual in nature. The phenomenon is not researched extensively but is clearly more common in adolescents.

WHAT IF WE WANT TO FIND OUT MORE?

Since men normally have erections during REM sleep, documentation of these nocturnal erections is the most likely way to find an erection if they exist at all. Until recently, their existence was assumed to rule out a physical cause and lead to the often-inaccurate diagnosis of psychogenic impotence.

Many men will be able to confirm the presence of morning erections based on their own observations. However, often they are not sure or don't notice. If not, there are a number of ways to assess **nocturnal penile tumescence (NPT).**

If the patient is not sure whether he's having a morning wake-up call, several tests can be used to document the event. A **snap gauge** is a device wrapped around the penis at bedtime that is held in place with a Velcro fastener. Different layers of the device rupture as a result of different erection forces during the night, leaving a trail of evidence regarding rigidity while asleep.

The snap gauge is easy to use, but its accuracy has been questioned. The greatest criticism is that it is easily tampered with if a patient wants to document an anatomic problem artificially instead of facing the fact that he has psychological rather than physical reason for his erectile dysfunction. The most likely motive for this tinkering would be in the now uncommon situation where a man's insurance plan requires documentation of physical abnormalities prior to covering further evaluation or treatment. Fortunately, most insurance companies have dropped these requirements based both on the consensus statements regarding erectile dysfunction and on the realization that these tests just added to their costs, usually without having an impact on further tests or treatments. Moreover, the snap gauge can also be forced open by a patient who can't allow himself to be judged incapable of having an erection.

A less expensive alternative to the snap gauge is to place a single layered coil of stamps around the penis before going to bed. When wrapped around the penis and stuck to itself the stamp band will rupture at the perforations if the penis becomes erect during the night. This is cheaper than the snap gauge, with price changes occurring only with congressional approval. The cost is dependent on the number of stamps required to encircle the penis, but don't let anyone know if you need fewer than three stamps to make it all the way around the shaft. Use of the stamps after testing is optional.

TESTING UNDER MEDICAL SUPERVISION

A more accurate and involved assessment of nocturnal erections can be obtained under physician supervision. Formal NPT testing can be done by using a complex measurement done in a sleep lab that gives more information than one could possibly ever need. The most elaborate testing occurs in a formal sleep laboratory using electroencephalography (EEG), electrooculography, and electromyography (EMG) to measure brain and other neurological activity. In addition, they measure nasal airflow and oxygen saturation to evaluate the severity of sleep apnea. Because readings during a so-called *first night effect* won't give a true picture of a man's sleep pattern, these tests are most accurate if performed over the course of two or three nights. Due to the cost and complexity, sleep lab studies are usually reserved for legal disability cases or as part of an overall sleep assessment for men with excessive snoring that are suspected to have **obstructive sleep apnea** (OSA, see chapter 6).

The **RigiScan** gives most of the same data at a fraction of the cost and can be done in the home setting. It allows portable monitoring in the comfort of your own bed. Before going to sleep, you place the ring's two loops around the base and tip of the penis in order to measure rigidity. Every three minutes during sleep, the loops constrict to a radial compression of 2.8 N.

If the base unit detects an increase in circumference greater than ten millimeters, the cycle speeds up to every thirty seconds. After three nights, the unit is returned to the physician for interpretation.

The greatest drawback of the RigiScan is that there is no universally accepted value of normal. Therefore this information must be considered as part of an overall assessment of the patient.

The fact that the penis expands doesn't necessarily mean that it is stiff enough to penetrate. Consequently, some authorities recommend awakening the man when the RigiScan indicates a maximal erection in order to check its quality. This can be done by taking a photograph or videotape, but the surest confirmation requires the placement of a device onto the tip of the penis to measure the weight required to bend it down (the "buckling strength"). If it can hold 1.5 kg (a little over three pounds), it should be able to penetrate the vagina.

NPT testing is believed to be the gold standard for documenting that a man is capable of having an erection on his own. A nocturnal erection requires intact nerves to the penis, normal blood flow, and indicates (although doesn't prove) that he has adequate hormones to have an erection. Still, most men don't need to be told their penis doesn't get hard at night, so most of this is usually not needed.

DOPPLER VASCULAR ASSESSMENT: WHEN YOU HAVE TO BE SURE

A **Doppler ultrasound** is a machine that has a probe that can be placed over an artery to confirm that it has flow inside. As a man achieves an erection, a Doppler will show colored flow in the artery in much the same way that the Doppler radar on the Weather Channel shows airflow in a tornado. This *Doppler effect* can be used to assess penile blood flow in cases where we must know.

The simplest setting to assess this flow is during an erection induced by *vibrotactile* or *audiovisual sexual stimulation* (*AVSS*). In layman's terms, that means an erection induced by some combination of masturbation, a vibrator, and viewing of an erotic videotape. This method is rarely used for obvious reasons. First, these activities and accoutrements may be acceptable in the privacy of one's own home, but aren't the typical activities of a doctor's office. It is difficult to not have the process feel "dirty" to the patient. Second, the office setting can be "castrating," and the stress of being in a relatively public setting may cause enough performance anxiety that an erection may not be representative of what a man is capable of anyway.

This technique was used inappropriately in the past to identify homosexual tendencies. Some men were subjected to testing to determine if they developed erections during the viewing of homoerotic material. We now know that a demonstration of erection, or the lack thereof, in this setting is not predictive of sexual orientation. Even if it were, the demonstration of arousal would not confirm that they acted on these tendencies and therefore was certainly not useful in making judgments such as whether they were suitable for military service based on laws prohibiting homosexuality.

A more reliable, and therefore more commonly used, test is to inject the **vasodilator** alprostadil into the penis. This opens the arteries irrespective of sexual stimulation and allows Doppler measurement of penile blood flow. Manual self-stimulation is sometimes added to assure that maximum flow is obtained. **Alprostadil** is one of several agents available to treat erectile dysfunction when injected into the penile shaft, as described in chapter 13.

Anxiety in the office setting can still be powerful enough to overcome alprostadil injection, so these studies must be interpreted with that in mind. However, Doppler ultrasound is the best study available at this time to confirm that penile blood flow is normal.

Another limitation of Doppler is in the natural arterial activity during an erection. Recall that arterial flow rises rapidly while the penis is filling. Once an erection is obtained, flow is actually fairly low, as the blood inside the corpora cavernosae is trapped under pressure. Therefore if Doppler measurement is made after the erection is complete, it may underestimate adequacy of arterial flow. The presence of a rock-hard erection should lead the interpreter to question any results that imply limited arterial flow.

In fact, if arterial flow is high during a full erection, it may indicate that the venous valves are not functioning properly; they may be allowing blood flow to exit the penis too quickly, which can indicate **venous insufficiency**. This can be quantified by a *resistive index*, which measures how much resistance the blood overcomes on its way through the penis. A low resistive index combined with a short-lived erection following alprostadil injection is a sure sign of venous insufficiency.

UNCOMMONLY USED TESTS

Several methods have been used historically to assess penile blood flow. They are described below mainly to inform the reader of their existence. Some physicians may still use them, but their limitations have made them uncommon.

The original method to assess adequacy of blood flow to the penis was the measurement of the *penile brachial pressure index (PBI)*. This compares the blood pressure in the penis to that of the rest of the body as indicated by the typical reading in the arm (hence "brachial"). Impaired penile blood flow was indicated by penile blood pressure less than 70 percent that of the systemic blood pressure. This was never very accurate for several reasons, the most significant of which is the difficulty in getting a correct blood pressure reading in the penis. Think about it—a pediatric blood pressure cuff was inflated around the shaft and someone listened to the tip of the penis using a stethoscope. A Doppler ultrasound machine could more accurately listen to penile blood flow during cuff inflation with improved accuracy. This test never had enough clinical utility to stand the test of time.

Penile plethysmography was a similar test that used a pediatric blood pressure cuff to constrict the penile arteries (and the entire penile shaft, for that matter). The cuff was then slowly deflated until blood flow returned. Its accuracy never justified its complexity, so the test is largely of historical significance.

Dynamic infusion cavernosometry and cavernosography (DICC) is a measurement of the ability of the penile sinusoids and veins to hold blood inside. It is an invasive measure used to quantify venous insufficiency. A needle is used to infuse the **corporal bodies** with a saline solution (sterile salt water) and measure how well it stays inside. An alprostadil injection assures blood flow is maximized as well. **Cavernosography** is the radiographic imaging done simultaneously. If venous insufficiency is present, it can demonstrate enlarged veins full of radiographic dye (or contrast) exiting the penis. If a single bad vein is identified, it can occasionally be tied off as described in chapter 15. Unfortunately, this test is invasive, difficult to perform, and more difficult to interpret. Therefore it is rarely performed, and normally only when someone is believed to be a serious candidate for **venous ligation surgery**.

Arteriography is used to confirm injury to the **pudendal arteries** leading into the penis. It is also discussed in chapter 15.

Cavernosal biopsy is a minor surgical procedure to remove and test a small piece of corporal tissue for abnormalities of nitric oxide synthetase or other enzymes involved in erections. Some surgeons recommend that the corporeal tissue be confirmed normal prior to vascular surgery, but this test is primarily used at this point for research.

Neurological tests to determine whether the nerves are properly hooked up are rarely needed. The most common is called *biothesiometry*. This test employs vibrations to assess nerve damage. Its accuracy is questioned because, although vibration may be a commonly used stimulation for females, it is not for males. In addition, defining "normal" is difficult. More involved neurological testing involves either *sacral evoked response, geneticerebral evoked potential studies,* or *dorsal nerve conduction velocity.* All three of these tests are needed uncommonly and mentioned for the purpose of completeness only.

In summary, several diagnostic tests have come and gone. For most men with erectile dysfunction, they are of historical interest only.

CHARLATANS AND QUACKS

The functional form of impotence fills the coffers of the quacks.
—Rutherford Morison, 1965

Before the introduction of Viagra, most men with erectile dysfunction went untreated. Physicians by nature don't take great interest in conditions that they can't help. Since impotence was believed to be entirely "in the head" in the vast majority of cases, most doctors didn't feel there was anything they could do to help. With millions of men suffering from erectile dysfunction, there was a huge void waiting to be filled. You could guess that someone would.

Many "men's health" centers arose in the late twentieth century, specializing in profitable evaluation and management of impotent men. Most were manned by nonurologists who were far better businessmen than physicians. They were typically discreetly placed, and they catered to the huge numbers of men whose needs were not being met in the regular doctor's office. Patients learned of their availability either by word of mouth or discreet ads placed in the back of the sports section of the newspaper.

When men enrolled in these programs, they were often regarded as untapped sources of gold. There was no such thing as the goal-oriented approach—far from it. Contrary to the recommendations of the International Consultation on Erectile Dysfunction to minimize diagnostic testing for most men, the goal of most of these centers was to collect as much revenue as possible. Blood test panels of every chemical that could be measured were performed. Most patients underwent most, if not all, of the tests mentioned in this chapter. After several thousand dollars' worth of tests, men were given the diagnosis: "You have erectile dysfunction."

Recall our diagnosis of erectile dysfunction from the beginning of this chapter. These men didn't need these tests to know what they had, but after all these tests, there was clearly no doubt.

After these tests, men were usually offered testosterone replacement, **vacuum constriction devices** (see chapter 11), or **intracorporeal pharmacotherapy** (see chapter 13). These options were appropriate, but the tests weren't required to know that.

Unfortunately, patients in these clinics weren't exactly in a position to shop around. Most regular physicians didn't have anything to offer them. Moreover, erectile dysfunction wasn't something that was discussed openly. Therefore, once inside closed doors, these men were essentially at the mercy of the proprietors.

Some of these men suffered complications from the treatments offered. Since the prescribing physicians were not formally trained in the methods, they usually weren't capable of handling complications like priapism or **fibrosis** (see chapter 13). Better businessmen than physicians, they therefore typically told their patients to go to a urologist or the emergency department of a local hospital if complications occurred. The courtesy of a call on behalf of their clients to a urologist was not part of the deal.

Urologists recognized the ethical outrage that was occurring and took a public stance against such endeavors in the nineties. As a result, the policy statement of the Sexual Medicine Society of North America is still included in the position statement of the American Urological Association. It concludes: "Ethical medical practice requires that diagnostic, therapeutic, and other decisions be made solely for the benefit of the patient and must be made without regard for the benefit of the health care provider" (this document can be found at the AUA Web site, www.ananet.org).

Fortunately, most of these centers have closed. The overriding reason for their demise was the sudden availability of oral therapy for erectile dysfunction. After the media blitz of Viagra's launch, it became acceptable for men to discuss erectile dysfunction. Men found out that they weren't alone. In addition, most physicians became aware of the scope of impotence in society and became comfortable in discussing it with patients and recommending treatment or consultation with a urologist. The cash cow for these centers disappeared.

KEY POINTS

- The American Urological Association and the 1992 NIH Consensus Statement define erectile dysfunction as "the inability to achieve or maintain an erection sufficient for satisfactory sexual performance."
- *Primary* impotence means that a man has never been able to achieve an erection. Most cases are *secondary*, occurring only after having normal erections previously.
- *Erectile dysfunction* is the preferred term for *impotence*. The latter term is less favored these days from a politically correct standpoint but remains the most common term for most people.
- The *goal-oriented approach* is appropriate for most men with erectile dysfunction. In cases that don't appear straightforward, or if a man feels it is imperative to know the cause, further testing is sometimes performed.
- A brief medical history and physical examination are adequate for most patients. Sexual questionnaires like the IIEF or SHIM can help quantify how much difficulty a man is having.
- Measurement of testosterone is usually performed, but involved tests of vascular status and neurological testing are rarely conducted.
- Differentiating between physical and psychological causes is useful, but most cases involve a little of both. The presence of nocturnal erections indicates that a man has at least some ability to have an erection.

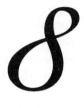

It Takes Two to Tango
Female Sexuality

Women and men are different.

—Anonymous

ccurately portraying the sexual male—as is attempted in the other chapters of this book—is a daunting task. At least it seems so until an attempt is made at portraying the sexual female. This task, in comparison, is monumental.

Whereas men, in general, can be lumped together with the widespread notion that most of them think of sex every eight seconds, women's sexuality is more varied. Some women have very little sex drive, while others make a longshoreman seem tame. In addition, when a man has erectile dysfunction, it's obvious what that means. On the contrary, female sexual dysfunction can mean anything from desire disorders to painful intercourse, with many other levels in between.

THE FEMALE ROLE IN
MALE ERECTILE DYSFUNCTION

[The bride] should be told that it is right and proper for her to experience pleasure in [sexual] performance.... It is only fair for the girl to understand that there is no immodesty in her active participation,

but on the contrary that such action on her part will increase the interest of the event for both her husband and herself.
—Denslow Lewis, "The Gynecologic Consideration of the Sexual Act," 1899

Sam Parker was a lucky guy. His internist found a minimally elevated **PSA** value during a routine physical exam when he was fifty. The PSA is a blood test used to detect **prostate** cancer (see chapter 3). A minimal elevation such as that found in Sam's blood work is sometimes a false alarm, but in this case, it turned out to be an early warning sign of prostate cancer. Having cancer can't be construed as lucky, but if you have it, finding out while it's still curable is certainly fortunate. At his age, Sam's best option involved **radical retropubic prostatectomy (RRP)** to remove the cancerous prostate.

Recall that prostate surgery can cause erectile dysfunction in some men due to injury to the nerves that go to the penis (chapter 2). Sam was concerned about this possibility, but was not taking any chances. He agreed with his girlfriend, Connie, that surgery should be scheduled.

The operation was successful. Both penile nerves were preserved, and the **biopsies** had shown that the cancer was confined to his prostate. With no spread of cancer, it was almost certain that the cancer was cured. He left the hospital the day after surgery and was back at work within four weeks as a metalworker. Indeed, he was a lucky guy.

At his appointment a month after surgery, Sam asked when it would be allowed to attempt intercourse. I reassured him that he could try anytime he desired, but I also warned him that most men will have a temporary period of erectile dysfunction even if the nerves are preserved and will eventually recover full function. Since he was very attracted to his younger girlfriend, he was motivated to try.

During the next follow-up visit three months later, Sam said that his penis was partially erect with stimulation, but he requested Viagra to help him achieve a full erection. He said he could penetrate with great effort, but that neither he nor Connie found it satisfying. I let them know that it usually takes several months after prostatectomy before Viagra seems to work fully (see chapter 12). This was to make sure they didn't put too much pressure on too soon. They both understood and confirmed a desire to try oral therapy.

During the year following surgery, Sam recovered fully and everything seemed great. On each visit he stated that they were sexually active about once a week and that he was satisfied with the quality of erections. The

Viagra helped make erection quality better, but even when he didn't take it, they were able to complete intercourse.

At the one-year visit, I congratulated Sam on his first of what I was confident would be many cancer-free years. We discussed all the issues that men face in recovering from prostate cancer, and he was upbeat about every topic except sex. I was concerned and reassured him that if erections weren't adequate, other treatments were available.

That's when he conceded that most of the issues recently had been with Connie and not with erectile dysfunction. She had undergone a hysterectomy a few months before. After that, she had vaginal dryness and tenderness and found vaginal penetration painful. Both Connie and Sam suffered from mild depression, but Connie found that she couldn't achieve **orgasm** while taking antidepressants. She continued to have some minor vaginal discharge postoperatively that caused embarrassment. This made her self-conscious about cleanliness, and although Sam didn't even notice it, she couldn't relax due to this concern.

Finally, Connie had been so scared by the news reports warning of the dangers of *estrogen replacement therapy* (*ERT*) that she stopped the hormone pills her gynecologist had prescribed to help with her symptoms. The dryness had subsequently gotten so bad that she winced whenever Sam tried to initiate sexual contact. That certainly didn't help his erections.

Sexual intercourse is always a two-person event. It is easy to focus on the man when a couple complains of erectile dysfunction, but part of his sexual response depends on interactions with his partner.

The most significant issue is in regard to how the woman responds to a sexual advance. Even a man with a completely normal erection otherwise will have a hard time keeping it up in the face of an unreceptive partner. This problem becomes magnified in a man whose erections are on the borderline.

A common scenario involves a couple that struggles with erectile dysfunction throughout the year, but has great sex while out of town on a relaxed vacation. Away from the stresses and responsibilities of home, it is not uncommon that the woman becomes more interested in sex. In contrast to the times at home when she sighs and consents to his advances in order to keep the peace, she may actually have a greater **libido** in the relaxed setting of vacation and may initiate sex herself. Assuming the man finds her approach stimulating, his borderline erections will probably need no other encouragement than her assertiveness. However, once they return home to the same old routine, the patterns frequently reemerge.

The partner should ideally be involved in any complex discussions regarding erectile dysfunction. She often has a different interpretation about what is going on. The erection he describes as being "a little bit soft" may be "useless" in the eyes of the partner. She may clarify that his statement regarding duration of erectile dysfunction should have been listed in years instead of weeks. Finally, she may throw in the "did he tell you about . . . ?" line regarding problems in the marriage or other issues that may play a role. Therefore the partner doesn't have to be involved in every patient encounter but may need to become involved if the man doesn't respond quickly to appropriate therapy.

As it turns out, Sam remains a lucky guy. Connie was concerned enough about her problems that she asked her gynecologist again about estrogen replacement. After starting the prescription, she regained libido and the pain ended. Orgasm became easier when she no longer needed the antidepressant. Their sex life is now satisfactory to them both. Even better, Sam's cancer appears to be cured.

WHAT A MAN NEEDS

> The solitude at night in bed is so depressing.
> —Johann Wolfgang von Goethe (1749–1832)

When a man begins having erectile dysfunction, his partner has three main options. The first and most common is to pretend not to notice. Only when the man brings it up does she say something like, "I barely noticed, although now that you mention it . . . but that's all right, dear." The second and more productive option is for the woman to express understanding and support, stating that the erection is adequate for her needs (if that is true), but that if he wants help in obtaining a better erection she will support him in that endeavor.

The final and disastrous reaction is for the woman to get upset. This can take one of two forms. The first is to assume that he doesn't find her attractive any longer. Maybe a little weight gain or a few wrinkles make her believe that she is less appealing than before. Her ego can then easily spiral downward, shaking her confidence in her own sex appeal. That will make her less likely to be sexually assertive, which means the man will be less stimulated. As you may guess, this doesn't help much. The second interpretation she might make is that the man isn't attracted to her because he's expending his sexual energies elsewhere. She may think he's cheating on her, and you could also guess that the stress of that interaction would not help him achieve a better erection.

The man's needs in this setting are optimally for the woman to provide support and understanding. This means avoiding the traps of believing that the man is cheating or doesn't find his mate attractive. I meet with many men about these issues, and a lack of desire for his partner is rarely in play. More likely, he desires his partner immensely but can't act upon his impulses. If the partner is putting these pressures on, it only makes it worse. They then have a problem that may need counseling or more aggressive intervention.

WHAT A WOMAN NEEDS

> Although physical sexual pleasure is not attached exclusively, or in the woman chiefly, to the act of coition [intercourse], it is a well-established fact that in healthy loving women ... increasing physical satisfaction attaches to the ultimate physical expression of love. A repose and general well-being results from this natural occasional intercourse, whilst the total deprivation of it produces irritability.
> —Elizabeth Blackwell, "The Human Element in Sex," 1902

It's easy to focus on the man's needs when he experiences erectile dysfunction, but the woman's needs are no less important. The woman's needs in this setting revolve around two issues. First and foremost is providing her with the security of knowing that her understandable fears are unfounded. She needs to know that her mate loves her and desires her. That doesn't mean she should be deluded into believing she is the most desirable woman who ever walked the earth. She just needs to know that she is the most desirable woman in the eyes of her mate. Interestingly, this is usually the case.

She needs to know that his erectile dysfunction is not her fault. Believing so would be no more accurate than believing that erectile dysfunction is usually due to psychological issues. On the contrary, just as we know that most cases of erectile dysfunction are due to physical causes, she needs to accept that this is the case and help her mate deal with erectile dysfunction in the same way she would accept and help him were he to come down with diabetes. Most importantly, she needs the security of knowing that his goal is retaining intimacy with her.

The second need of the woman is her own sexual satisfaction. This is more complex than it appears, since neither partner may have a definitive idea of what that entails. Many women aren't set in their own expectations, so how would men who certainly can't read their minds be expected to know what they are?

Many men get it in their minds that sex doesn't count unless it includes an orgasm. This is true in the minds of men, but not necessarily so in the minds of women. About one-fourth of women never have an orgasm, and few women reach orgasm each time they have sex.[1] That means that disappointment will be common if the man expects he will bring his mate to orgasm each time they have intercourse. That expectation is a setup for failure. In contrast to men, orgasm may not be the ultimate goal for women. Instead, their goal is sometimes simply intimacy or other pleasures of sex that don't necessarily involve orgasm.

The most important thing for the couple to do is to communicate their needs to each other as well as they can. If orgasm isn't important to the woman, she should reassure her husband that her needs don't necessarily include it. Then, they can focus on what their needs really are. The intimacy may be what each of them needs the most, and this may or may not have to include vaginal penetration. If not, some couples discover that intercourse isn't the real goal, so treatment becomes very easy.

If penetration is the goal, then making sure the man can do so becomes the focus. If orgasm of the female partner is the goal, then it is essential to determine what makes her most likely to do so. Few women have orgasm solely based on vaginal penetration, so foreplay involving stimulation of the female partner (especially the **clitoris**) may need to be expanded. A female partner who can communicate this need combined with a male partner who is willing to do whatever it takes to satisfy his partner is the most likely combination for success.

FEMALE ERECTILE DYSFUNCTION?

> I'll have what she's having.
> —Meal order taken from the woman sitting near Sally in
> *When Harry Met Sally*, following Sally's very public
> demonstration of a convincing fake orgasm

Sexual dysfunction in a man is tangible. It involves a visible demonstration—the penis is unable to perform. However, women with sexual dysfunction can still perform as long as they are capable of lying still. Even without any interest in intercourse, a woman can allow vaginal penetration and complete intercourse. Whereas a man can't fake an erection any more than a wet noodle can pry open a deadbolt, a motivated woman can fake the whole thing. Anyone who saw Meg Ryan's famous restaurant scene in *When Harry Met Sally* can attest to the fact that a fake orgasm is easy to carry off for a woman. This is unique to women—most men can't fathom why anyone would fake an orgasm.

However, the female version of erectile dysfunction is *female sexual dysfunction*. This term encompasses a wide range of female sexual dissatisfactions. To sort them out, the *Sexual Function Health Council* of the American Foundation of Urological Diseases in 1998 brought together nineteen experts in sexual dysfunction. Specialists in urology, psychiatry, gynecology, endocrinology, family medicine, nursing, pharmacology, psychology, and rehabilitation medicine were assembled to define and classify female sexual dysfunction. This was the first large-scale attempt to look seriously at an area that prior to that time had been mostly ignored. They defined *female sexual dysfunction* as comprising several subcategories of conditions that caused personal distress. These included *hypoactive sexual desire disorder* (diminished libido), *sexual aversion disorder* (avoidance and actual phobia of sexual contact), *sexual arousal disorder* (physical abnormalities that impair normal vaginal changes during arousal), and *orgasmic disorder* (inability to achieve orgasm).

Another definition is in the *Diagnostic and Statistical Manual IV*. This book, usually referred to as *DSM-IV*, is the bible of diagnostic definitions and defines the terminology most commonly used by psychiatrists and other mental health professionals. It defines sexual dysfunction as a "disturbance in sexual desire and in the psychophysiological changes that characterize the sexual response cycle and cause marked distress and interpersonal difficulty."

The classification of diseases according to the World Health Organization's (WHO), named *ICD-10*, defines sexual dysfunction as including "the various ways in which an individual is unable to participate in a sexual relationship as he or she would wish." These definitions therefore describe various forms of female sexual dysfunction, as well as male erectile dysfunction.

Painful intercourse is called **dyspareunia**. It can be due to physical abnormalities such as vaginal pain or inflammation, but is often due to **vaginismus** or involuntary spasms of the pelvic and vaginal muscles as a conditioned response to problems that would make the woman wish to avoid intercourse. This is another of those **vicious cycles** that occur when one problem perpetuates another, while the second starts the process over again. An initial discomfort with intercourse can progress into severe spasms and pain if allowed to continue. Thereafter, each time a penis comes close, the vaginal and pelvic floor muscles clamp down and make it just that much more unlikely for the problem to be solved.

PARALLELS OF FEMALE SEXUAL DYSFUNCTION AND MALE ERECTILE DYSFUNCTION

> Sex is metaphysical for men, as it is not for women. Women have no problems to solve through sex.
> —Camille Paglia, *Sexual Personae*, 1990

The parallels of female sexual function disorder and male erectile dysfunction are intriguing. Recall that over half of all men will suffer from erectile dysfunction at some point in their lives. Although surveys of women have not been as complete, it appears that the same percentage of women suffer female sexual function disorder. The National Health and Social Life Survey found that 43 percent of women *below the age of sixty* had complaints of sexual dysfunction.[2] Knowing that women continue to report increasing sexual difficulties with aging, we can extrapolate that at least half of women will suffer them at some point in their lifetimes.

In addition, the risk factors for female sexual dysfunction mirror those for male erectile dysfunction. These include most of the issues discussed for men in chapter 6, including aging, hypertension (high blood pressure), smoking, high cholesterol, and pelvic surgery. Therefore, it could be said that female sexual dysfunction is the female analog of male erectile dysfunction.

NORMAL FEMALE SEXUAL RESPONSE

As with men, there really is no such thing as "normal" female sexual behavior. Interpretation of the sights, sounds, smells, and touches that comprise potentially erotic stimuli varies by the beholder. How one reacts to those stimuli definitely varies. However, we do know with reliability some changes that occur with sexual stimulation.

Masters and Johnson observed women as well as men. They divided sexual response into the same four phases described for men in chapter 4. The *excitement* phase in women begins with engorgement of the vaginal tissues, leading to excretion of lubricating fluid. The vagina elongates and the clitoris fills. The *plateau* phase involves an increase in these changes, along with a quickening of the pulse. The clitoris almost disappears beneath the hood of tissue overlying it due to engorgement of that tissue.

During the third phase, *orgasm*, physical pleasure maximizes, augmented with the rhythmic contractions of the vaginal, pelvic, and other nearby skeletal muscles causing pelvic thrusting at intervals of over once per second. These female muscular contractions can be the most stimulating event during intercourse for men, sometimes causing the man to cross an orgasmic threshold as well. The uterus contracts while heart rate and blood pressure reach their peaks. Finally, the *resolution* phase occurs as heart rate and blood pressure return to normal, while the vascular congestion of the pelvic tissues resolves.

Obviously, women frequently have intercourse without going through all four phases. Although the concept of a simultaneous orgasm in men and women is celebrated in the media, it is actually very uncommon for men and women to both reach satisfaction at the exact same moment. Due to the refractory period men experience immediately following orgasm (see chapter 4, "Orgasm: The Ultimate Goal?"), attempting to might not be worth it for most couples. If the man ejaculates even seconds before his mate reaches climax, he may find the muscular contractions of her orgasm to be an unpleasant conclusion to intercourse. The woman probably won't notice a difference, as the penis will usually stay rigid during the remaining seconds of her orgasm.

UNDERSTANDING THE VAGINA

The female sex organs all relate in some way to the vagina in a manner similar to the way secondary sex organs in a male relate to the penis. The female pelvic anatomy can be broken down into two categories—internal and external. The external anatomical organs are collectively known as the **vulva**, and include the labia (the "lips" on either side), the clitoris, and some minor glands. The *labia majora* are the thick hair-bearing folds on the thigh side, whereas the *labia minora* are the hairless, thinner folds on the vaginal side. The *internal genitalia* include *the ovaries, the uterus, the fallopian tubes*, and most of the *vagina* (see Fig. 3).

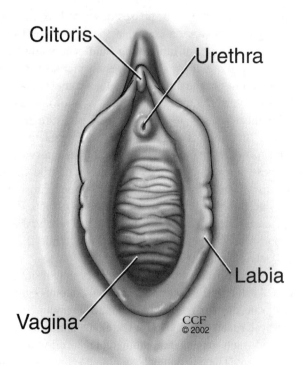

Fig. 3. Female anatomy.

The vagina is a soft cylinder that serves as the route from the uterus to the outside world (for menstrual flow or delivery of a baby) as well as the route from the outside world into the uterus and fallopian tubes (for **semen** to perpetuate the species). The vagina is actually a pretty tough organ, comprised of three strong layers supported by a rich tree of nerves and blood vessels responsible for engorgement during sexual stimulation.

Although it appears to be a round tube, we know that the vagina in cross section is really shaped more like the letter H unless something is holding it open. The nerves that allow pleasurable sexual stimulation are primarily in the outer third of the vagina, making it possible for a man with any size penis to be satisfying (see chapter 2, "Does size really matter?"). This finding has led many people to theorize the existence of the G-spot, which was described in 1982 by German gynecologist Dr. Ernst Grafenberg. This magical spot on the anterior wall of the vagina is said to hold the key to female stimulation. Unfortunately, no one has ever been able to demonstrate this structure anatomically. Therefore, it appears that pleasurable sensations of the anterior vaginal wall are simply due to the high concentration of nerves in that location combined with the blood flow that increases with arousal. The Grafenberg spot appears to be nonexistent, although the anterior vaginal wall in that area is naturally more stimulating than surrounding tissues for many women.

Sexual arousal initiates increased blood flow into the vagina and clitoris in a manner similar to what occurs during a normal erection in a man. The increased blood flow causes lubricating fluid to cross its walls. The *vestibular* or *Bartholin's glands* also help produce lubricating fluid. They are also thought by some experts to have a more primal purpose in producing scents to attract the male partner in a manner similar to pheromones (see chapter 10, "The five senses").

The pelvic floor muscles are more critical in a woman than in a man for a couple of reasons. Importantly to our topic, rhythmic contractions of the pelvic floor muscles are responsible for much of the pleasurable sensations experienced during female orgasm. During intercourse, these muscles are also responsible for the vagina shortening and lengthening during stimulation. This action is equally important for enjoyment of the partner, as these contractions are powerfully stimulating to most men.

Problems associated with the pelvic floor muscles include either weakness or pain. If either the bladder (*cystocele*) or rectum (*rectocele*) pushes the weakened vaginal wall into the tubular space of the vagina, they can protrude out through the vaginal opening. These are not perceptible to either partner during intercourse, so only cause sexual problems in rare, severe cases. These conditions rarely cause pain and have to be surgically corrected only if symptomatic.

Finally, uncontrolled contractions of these muscles can cause the painful, uncontrolled spasms of vaginismus.

THE FEMALE PHALLUS

The **clitoris** is the female version of a penis. That doesn't mean it is like a penis—it *is* a penis. During fetal development, the primitive *genital tubercle* arises as three cylinders that eventually develop into either the penis or clitoris. The three cylinders become an obvious phallic structure if the fetus develops into a male, comprised of the paired **corpora cavernosae** and the single **corpus spongiosum** (as described in chapter 2).

Much to the surprise of most men and women alike, these same three structures are present in the female clitoris. Just like the penis, the clitoral cavernosal bodies separate to attach to the ischial bones inside the pelvis. The inner length is similar to that of the penis but simply stops at the skin level instead of protruding outside the body wall as the penis does. The clitoral *glans* (called *glans clitoris* instead of **glans penis**) is the only part that usually makes it outside skin level in a woman. Therefore, the portion of the clitoris that is visible (or can be felt) is the glans clitoris. The clitoris lacks the strong **tunica albuginea** of the penis, so it can't trap blood inside for a full erection. That means that during the time blood flow in the clitoris doubles due to sexual stimulation, it achieves engorgement instead of erection. However, just as the glans penis is the most sensitive and pleasurable part of the male anatomy, the glans clitoris is the most sensitive and pleasurable part of the female anatomy. Therefore, most women experience enough stimulation to achieve orgasm mainly with clitoral stimulation—not vaginal.

NITRIC OXIDE IN THE WOMAN? NO WAY!

Many of the activities that occur in the vagina during sexual stimulation are controlled by **nitric oxide**. Yes, the same *neurotransmitter* (abbreviated **NO**, discussed in chapter 4, "NO way") that was responsible for the chemical cascade resulting in the male erection. Are you noticing a pattern of the parallels of women and men? Another neurotransmitter involved is *vasointestinal peptide* (*VIP*), which has been used to create erections by direct injection into the penis (see chapter 13, "Newer drugs"). Nitric oxide and VIP (potentially along with some other agents under investigation) have been shown to have several actions on the female sexual mechanism just as they have in men. This finding has led to intense interest in using oral medications developed for erectile dysfunction in an attempt to improve sexual function in women. Viagra has been shown in the laboratory setting to relax rabbit clitoral and vaginal tissues, which would indicate that it should help improve sexual function. VIP also appears to have the same effect, as well as causing enhanced vaginal blood flow, lubrication, and secretions. Several trials of Viagra have shown improved sexual function in some women, as discussed later in this chapter.

THE ROLE OF HORMONES IN FEMALE SEXUAL FUNCTION

Hormones appear to be more important in female sexual function than they are in men. That includes the female hormone estrogen, and to the surprise of many, it also includes the male hormone **testosterone**. That doesn't seem to make sense—testosterone makes men desire women, right? Well, apparently it actually just makes humans (and other animals, for that matter) desire sexual activity.

The best evidence of this fact is in the testosterone surge that premenopausal women have during the middle of their menstrual cycles. This coincides with the time when they are maximally fertile, so it makes sense that nature would make women more likely to desire intercourse during this fertility peak. Women are indeed most sensuous during this portion of the menstrual cycle, confirming the theory. The surge of testosterone appears to be that stimulus.

It makes sense that sexual activity is most enjoyable during the reproductive years, since survival of the species depends on it. Therefore the hormones involved in libido decrease with aging after they are no longer needed to assure procreation. Testosterone levels are cut in half by the time women reach their forties. Fortunately, menopause doesn't make these levels fall significantly further. However, surgical removal of the ovaries essentially stops testosterone production. Therefore, testosterone replacement may be most important for women who have had this operation, as discussed below. Finally, sensation is measurably impaired in the setting of inadequate estrogen, obviously leading to decreased pleasure with sex.

Another hormone that appears to be critical in female sexual response is DHEA. Women with DHEA levels below normal have significantly more sexual complaints than those with normal levels. Companies that make nutritional supplements have touted DHEA as a cure-all for male or female sexual problems. However, there is little scientific evidence on such supplements (as discussed in chapter 11).

Some researchers have indicated that long-term (many years) oral contraceptive use may hurt the female hormonal apparatus. It has been shown that women on birth control pills have statistically decreased libido compared to women who don't use oral contraceptives. In addition, the midcycle testosterone surge that is responsible for improved libido during peak fertility is blunted by birth control pills.

OTHER CAUSES OF FEMALE SEXUAL DYSFUNCTION

The overlap of causes of female sexual dysfunction and male erectile dysfunction is manifold. As noted above, low testosterone levels decrease libido in men and women. In addition, anything that impairs blood flow to the female genitalia will cause problems. This can be due to **arteriosclerosis** or injuries to the arteries through surgery or smoking. Pelvic fractures or bicycling injuries can affect women's genital blood flow just as they do in men.

Injury to the pelvic nerves from prostate surgery is known to cause male erectile dysfunction. Similarly, women with anything that harms the pelvic nerves risk sexual dysfunction. Common causes include pelvic surgery, diabetes, multiple sclerosis, or spinal cord injuries. These conditions are especially pronounced in regard to orgasm, as it appears that orgasm is largely a spinal reflex.

A list of medications that can cause erectile dysfunction is included in chapter 6. Many of these medications have been reported to cause female sexual side effects as well. Especially important in women are drugs (such as cimetidine, spironolactone, or ketoconazole) that affect hormones. Birth control pills and treatments for breast cancer such as tamoxifen can directly inhibit hormone production.

Many chronic diseases are associated with female sexual dysfunction. Diabetic women frequently report poor libido and difficulties achieving orgasm, perhaps related to diabetic nerve damage called *neuropathy*. Moreover, cancer of any kind will negatively affect health, but cancers specific to females may add the stigma of altered body image. Therefore, some women who have had removal of a breast or uterus may have feelings of diminished femininity, which may translate into sexual dysfunction. Rheumatoid arthritis, Crohn's disease, multiple sclerosis, and kidney failure are also known to cause sexual problems.

THE ROLE OF THE MIND
IN FEMALE SEXUAL DYSFUNCTION

If the male mind plays a major role in erections (recall that erectile dysfunction is not usually *only* in the mind, but it still plays a crucial part), the female mind plays an even greater role. Whereas many men desire sex as a way to feel intimacy, most women have sex *because* they feel intimacy. The relationship with the man and other emotional issues are almost always part of the picture. Women who feel diminished self-esteem or who suffer from a negative body image will have a difficult time relaxing enough to become aroused. This is commonly exhibited in the situation of a woman who doesn't feel as attractive as she used to, so she doesn't want to undress and reveal her inadequacies. Usually, her mate either doesn't care about these perceived inadequacies or simply doesn't see them. Therefore he simply feels shut out by her.

Any psychological condition can affect female sexuality. The most common one is depression. The catch-22 is that depression limits libido and causes female sexual dysfunction, and most medications used to treat depression inhibit orgasm. The prescriptions usually used for depression are called SSRI medications. Their side effect of impairing orgasm is actually used to treat men with rapid ejaculation (chapter 5, "Rapid relief with medications"). The impairment of orgasm isn't sought after among women, who typically have a more difficult time reaching orgasm to begin with. Therefore, a woman with poor libido might be treated with an SSRI, but once she is aroused enough to have intercourse, the very same drug might prevent her from having an orgasm. (Some studies have indicated that women who experience this may benefit from Viagra or other oral medications.[3] However, women who use Viagra with **nitrates** are at the same risk of death from combining it with nitrates that men are. These are fully discussed in chapter 12.)

EVALUATION OF FEMALE SEXUAL DYSFUNCTION

Women with sexual dysfunction often don't consider investigation. However, for those who do, several things can be measured. As hormones are more critical to female sexuality, measurement is taken of *follicle-stimulating hormone (FSH)*, *luteinizing hormone (LH)*, *prolactin*, *testosterone*, *sex hormone binding globulin*, and *estradiol*.

Initial evaluation in men usually involves checking whether the penis ever becomes erect. This finding is documentable (as discussed in chapter 7.) However, women may have significant physical findings such as impaired blood flow, elasticity, or lubrication that aren't easily observed. Some research centers are investigating genital blood flow using a duplex **Doppler ultrasound** in a manner like that used in men. Other investigational measures include *vaginal lubrication*, *vaginal compliance/elasticity*, *pressure/volume* changes, and genital *vibrational sensation*. These are not standardized and should be considered investigational at this time.

A brief psychological investigation should be part of any case where intervention is being considered. This should include the woman's overall mental health status as well as self-esteem, body image, and a woman's ability to communicate her sexual needs with her partner. A sexual function questionnaire like those described for men in chapter 7 has been validated for women. The *Brief Index of Sexual Function Inventory for Women* (*BISF-W*) is a 21-item inventory of sexual interest, activity, satisfaction, and preference that can assemble this information efficiently.

TREATMENT

Until now, the only treatments for female sexual complaints following menopause have been hormone replacement, lubricants, psychotherapy, and antidepressants. Just as men are best managed using the **goal-oriented approach**, women should be offered similar methodology.

The most effective treatments so far have involved testosterone replacement. Although there is no FDA-approved testosterone replacement for women, it is possible to replace testosterone using a pellet, pills, injections, skin creams, or patches, as is done in men. Studies have shown that women have improved libido, orgasmic potential, and overall well-being if testosterone is properly administered under the care of a physician. That usually means that the patients who should receive testosterone replacement are postmenopausal.

All male hormones (androgens) can cause *masculinization* or *virilization* in women. That means women can develop physical changes associated with male characteristics, like excessive hair growth or acne. Menstrual irregularities are common, and in cases of excessive testosterone administration, patients can develop male pattern baldness, voice changes, or clitoral growth (recall that the clitoris is just the penis that was never exposed to the hormones that would have made it grow). These changes are largely irreversible, so these treatments should be monitored closely. Finally, testosterone can be converted to estrogen in the body, so women with a history of breast cancer should not take testosterone replacement, as this can cause growth of the cancer.

The easiest way to give testosterone is by the oral medication called *methyl testosterone*. However, reports of liver damage in men taking oral testosterone must give caution. *Estratest* is a combination of methyl testosterone and estrogen that can be used orally to replace deficiency of both hormones.

Testosterone replacement is most important in women who have had the ovaries surgically removed. This is because testosterone production normally continues even after menopause has allowed estrogen production to subside. Therefore, postmenopausal women retain markedly greater levels of testosterone than women who have had both ovaries removed.

Estrogen replacement therapy received a lot of negative press in recent years due to reports that it might contribute to cancer or other serious diseases. There is some validity to the criticism, but this can also overshadow a legitimate need for physiological replacement. Simply giving hormones to women isn't logical, but restoring their levels to normal in order to treat symptoms as varied as sexual dysfunction, urinary incontinence, and pelvic pain from dryness should be weighed. In addition, treating osteoporosis and other systemic diseases due to estrogen deficiency can be lifesaving. Therefore, instead of making broad statements, patients should be treated as individuals.

The greatest risk of estrogen replacement therapy is in causing *endometrial cancer* of the uterus. This is due to estrogen being allowed to stimulate growth of the uterine lining continually, and can be prevented by giving progesterone intermittently to prevent over stimulation of the lining. They may be prescribed separately or as the combination of *Prempro*.

ON THE HORIZON

All other treatments for female sexual dysfunction are experimental at this writing, but some encouraging findings are emerging. After years of prejudice that female sexual dysfunction is "in the head," intense interest has led to research initiatives at major medical centers around the world. Again, note the parallel with the history of male erectile dysfunction.

Viagra is the most studied drug for female sexual dysfunction. Initial reports indicated no benefit, but in selected situations there is recent evidence that it may play a role. The primary use for Viagra (and theoretically, the other **phosphodiesterase [PDE] inhibitors**) is apparently to improve genital blood flow and sensation. It appears to improve libido and orgasm in women with spinal cord injury, postmenopausal women, and those using an SSRI as discussed above.

L-arginine is an *amino acid*—one of the essential building blocks of all proteins. It has been shown to improve erections in men with mild erectile dysfunction. It has been used in women in combination with **yohimbine** (see chapter 12) on an experimental basis.

Prostaglandin E1 is used in injectable treatment used in men with erectile dysfunction with great success, as discussed in chapter 13. The Vivus Corporation is currently investigating its use intravaginally for women, as well as the use of a drug called *TA-1790* that would be used in combination with it. They have received a patent (U.S. patent number 6,649,016) for the combination. TA-1790 is a phosphodiesterase inhibitor from the same group of drugs that includes Viagra and the newer oral medications for erectile dysfunction.

Another **vasodilator** similar to prostaglandin E1 is **phentolamine**. It is being investigated for use in both men and women. It has demonstrated enhanced vaginal blood flow and increased arousal in women in early trials. Finally, **apomorphine** is a drug that is available for erectile dysfunction in many countries as the brand name **Uprima** or *Ixense*. Approval for use in the United States met several obstacles due to side effects. It is used in animals to induce vomiting, so nausea is obviously a common side effect. It has not been fully studied in women at the time of this writing.

WHAT MEN/WOMEN NEED

Earlier in this chapter, we discussed the needs of each partner when a man experiences erectile dysfunction. This can be turned around when women have sexual dysfunction. In that setting, the man often feels that his partner is "frigid" or selfish. He may perceive that she is unwilling to meet his sexual needs. Feelings are easily hurt.

In contrast, the woman may feel pressured to have sex when she has no interest. Her lack of interest may not be related to relationship issues, and in fact, she may feel close to her partner in every other way. However, if she has no interest in sex, she will have a difficult time faking it. If problems achieving orgasm are the issue, some women *will* fake it, as Sally demonstrated in *When Harry Met Sally*.

A successful outcome will involve both partners feeling valued yet satisfied. Compromise will be necessary. If both partners are motivated to meet the needs of the other while strengthening the emotional bonds of their relationship, success should be achievable.

KEY POINTS

- Sexual relationships will always involve two disparate individuals with distinct needs.
- A man dealing with erectile dysfunction will be more likely to achieve success if his partner is supportive and cooperative. Likewise, a woman dealing with sexual dysfunction will be more likely to achieve success if her partner is supportive and cooperative.
- Female sexual dysfunction is remarkably similar to male erectile dysfunction. The causes and issues overlap substantially.
- Erectile dysfunction is easily recognizable, but female sexual dysfunction may exhibit no physical findings. Most cases involve interest in sex or orgasmic difficulties and not observable physical abnormalities.
- Restoring normal levels of estrogen can offer significant improvement in both libido and pleasure of intercourse for women.
- Testosterone replacement improves libido but must be prescribed with caution in order to avoid its masculinizing side effects.
- Women who have had surgical removal of the ovaries are especially likely to receive benefit from testosterone replacement.

9 Getting the Most from a Trip to the Urology Office

A urologist is another personality type altogether.
There's a civility and seriousness to urologists, but also a strange wryness. You have to tell them things you'd just as soon not tell yourself, and so the patients tend to speak in euphemisms: "Doc, I got a thing with my thing."
People who know doctors swear they can always spot the urologist. It's the lack of pomposity, but also the surety of ego. Stern, unfazed, methodical, frequently German, as if for effect.
—Hank Stuever, *Washington Post* Staff Writer

*T*here's an old joke that if someone finishes at the bottom of the medical school class, they call him "doctor." However, if he finishes near the top of his class despite everyone's impression that he isn't serious enough to do so, they may end up calling him "urologist." Urologists tend to be class clowns who seem to take everything lightly but somehow end up winning a competitive spot for one of medicine's "hot" specialties. Combining the academic standing required to make the cut with the personality suited to deal with peoples' most private issues, we are known as a unique, perhaps quirky, group.

Neurosurgeons are asked interesting questions about the origin of human thought or the neurobiological implications of the soul, while urologists are more likely to be asked, "Why would anyone want to do that for a living?" Urologists are admittedly a different breed. We spend our days doing things that would mortify our mothers. Most patients we meet drop their pants at some point in the conversation. That takes a little getting used to. We never get to experience "take your daughters to work day." Nevertheless, urologists are among the happiest and most highly regarded physicians, so it's worth it all.

If you are reading this book, it is likely you could end up in a urologist's office at some point. Therefore, the following pages will discuss the interactions you might expect.

GETTING READY FOR THE UROLOGY APPOINTMENT

No matter what reason brings you to the urology office, many of the basic experiences of patients overlap. You will probably be asked to fill out a detailed medical history form prior to seeing the doctor. This might be mailed before the appointment, or might be given to you upon arrival.

The information requested will be addressing two needs. The first need to be met is to find out why you are there and what your problem is. The second need is to fulfill requirements placed on physicians by Medicare and other insurers. These regulations require the collection and documentation of a lot of information that may seem medically unnecessary but must be charted in order to remain within federal guidelines.

The first question asks your *chief complaint*. Literally, this means, "Why are you here?" If erectile dysfunction is the concern, some patients will honestly report it. More common responses are evasive ones like "personal problems," "prostate problems," or "consultation." A straightforward, honest response when filling out the forms helps you get more from the visit, so try to be above board. Some patients write down fake concerns and only when asked if there is "anything else?" do they mumble something about erections under their breath. If the doctor doesn't probe for more information, the real concern could end up not being addressed at all.

Next, some general medical information will be gathered. Physicians traditionally group this information in standardized fashion, which is similar independent of specialty. Medicare began requiring that this information be documented in a standard format in the last decade. Although not all patients are on Medicare, it is the most influential economic force in health care. Therefore, this format will dictate information gathering at many office visits. The *past medical history* (*PMH*) and *past surgical history* (*PSH*) require listing of the illnesses, hospitalizations, and operations that have affected your present physical state. *Medications* and *allergies* are listed and flagged for future reference when it comes time to consider writing a prescription. An abbreviated *social history* asks about marital status, occupation, and tobacco or alcohol use. Finally, a *review of systems* will ask some simple questions about other body organ systems, from the neurological to the urological. This same information is obtained whether you have a weak heart, a weak knee, or a weak erection.

The questions asked about your specific complaint will address at least four of the following *qualifying factors*:

Location:	Where is the problem?
Duration:	How long has it bothered you?
Timing:	Is it constant or intermittent?
Quality:	How would you describe the symptoms?
Severity:	How bad is it?
Context:	In what situation does it occur?
Modifying factors:	Have you had previous treatment?
Associated symptoms:	Anything else you notice that's wrong?

Assuming a visit for erectile dysfunction, we can answer all eight *qualifying factors* easily.

Location:	Penis
Duration:	For a long time
Timing:	Bad
Quality:	Poor
Severity:	Severe enough to discuss with a professional
Context:	During sexual activity
Modifying factors:	I haven't done anything yet
Associated symptoms:	Angst!

After obtaining the above information, the doctor will explore the specific concern leading to this visit. In the example of erectile dysfunction, this might involve a conversation. Alternatively, the information might be obtained by a sexual history questionnaire as discussed in chapter 7. Many of these are commercially available and help assure that nothing is left out during an office visit. Many urologists have created their own forms to ask these questions in a manner that allows them to focus on the issues they feel are important for patients with erectile dysfunction. Some may not use questionnaires at all but may ask you direct questions that will contribute to their **goal-oriented approach** (chapter 7, "The goal-oriented approach").

CHECKING IN: BE PREPARED

Gordon arrived for his consultation regarding erectile dysfunction with Dr. Brown ten minutes after his scheduled appointment. He didn't have an insurance card or any information on how the visit was covered. He said that he took some medications prescribed by an internist, but he didn't know anything about them except their color and that they "cost too damned much." He knew he had an operation on his testicles when he was a teenager but didn't know why it was done. He was "deathly allergic" to some pill "that a quack doctor made me take," but he had no idea what it was or why he had even taken it. For that matter, he didn't know what side effect it caused—just that he was sure he was allergic to it. Despite his inability and unwillingness to supply any information except the fact that he "couldn't keep it up," he was ready for a diagnosis to be dished out and a prescription to be written within thirty seconds of sitting down in the office. More important things awaited back at *his* office.

When people go to see a movie, they come prepared. They know why they are there and which movie they want tickets for. They have money ready. If hungry, they go straight to the concession stand and order exactly what they want. They empty their bladder if they think the movie will take long enough to cause discomfort. My wife always remembers to bring a sweater, even in the summer, because the theater may be too cool.

If only people came to the doctor's office so well prepared. Many, like Gordon, come without having their necessary medical information available. They expect the doctor to make recommendations on their health care without providing the necessary information to do so. In Gordon's case, the pill that made him "deathly ill" was nitroglycerin. The reason he vomited the time he took it was that he was having a heart attack. He no longer used regular nitroglycerine, but took it daily in a sustained release form. He wasn't allergic—just clueless. The prescription he demanded without an examination or gathering of any history was for Viagra. Had this been dished out as requested, he could have easily died in bed later that night.

Fortunately for Gordon, Dr. Brown did his homework before fulfilling his demands.

When checking into any doctor's office these days, you should know your insurance status. Your insurance may not pay for any of the visit or tests obtained unless preapproved. Ignorance of this policy won't remove your financial responsibility, so get ready to pay if you don't find out. Their policy regarding prescription drugs will play a role in what medications you might take and what quantity should be prescribed. If they would pay for a ninety-day supply of medications, you should know that before paying the same amount (*co-pay*) for a thirty day supply. If they cover one drug instead of another equivalent drug, you'll want to let the doctor know so he can decide if the suggested drug is an acceptable alternative (See a discussion of the importance of this in chapter 13, "When is generic more expensive?")

Some people take the approach that it's someone else's responsibility to keep up with their insurance status. Those are the people likely to be left responsible for the bill.

An inadequate medical history can yield disastrous results. If Dr. Brown had not figured out that Gordon took nitroglycerin, its interaction with Viagra could have been fatal. The failure to understand that one of his testicles had been removed for a tumor that caused hormonal abnormalities meant that the man was running on essentially no **testosterone**. The other testicle had burned out, so he was functionally a *eunuch*. Although we know that testosterone isn't absolutely required for an erection, it does play a role in the big picture as discussed in chapter 6. Fortunately, the doctor recognized this when the patient finally slowed down enough to have a simple examination. A prescription for testosterone replacement therapy solved the problem quickly and permanently—except that "it cost too damned much."

Upon check-in, give the necessary information to the office staff. Have your medical history information available and ready. If any tests have been performed prior to that time that are related to this visit, make sure to ask the staff to ensure that the results are on your chart instead of waiting until you are face to face with the doctor.

THE GENERAL EXAMINATION

Although an examination of the penis might be the only thing expected, remember that no penis is an island. The doctor will begin the examination before you probably even realize it. He will note your weight, build, and whether normal signs of *masculinization* are present. Certain body shapes are related to syndromes that might not cause serious health problems, but might affect erections. If these syndromes are suspected, more tests might be recommended.

The body of a weightlifter will make the doctor curious about steroid use. Later on, he will be especially observant of testicular size if he suspects you use steroids, as they may shrink the testicles to the size of marbles. Perfect pecs combined with tiny testicles will be a sure giveaway that steroid use is part of the problem.

The neck might be examined for thyroid abnormalities that could affect overall health and erections. A cursory heart and lung exam might be done to assure that the person is capable of having and using erections. An abdominal examination to check for tumors or hernias is part of a routine physical examination as well, although they don't directly affect erections. Finally, the blood pressure and pulse are checked to see if there is any severe systemic disease.

THE GENITAL EXAMINATION: DROP 'EM

Men love dropping their pants—except in the urologist's office. Suddenly, modesty abounds. Try to get over it. After all, the office visit is to help you drop 'em more often, so this temporary embarrassment is worth it.

The penis is examined for external lesions, or for signs of venereal diseases. The foreskin is retracted in uncircumcised men in order to assure there are no tumors and to assess the health of the **glans penis**. The shaft is *palpated* deeply by squeezing it between fingers to check for **Peyronie's** plaques (see chapter 7).

The testicles are examined mainly for size and tumors. Small gonads indicate that low testosterone might be part of the problem. If they appear large, it is usually due to fluid around them. This fluid might be a small collection of sperm (called a *spermatocele*) or just body fluid (called a *hydrocele*). A collection of *varicose veins* in the **scrotum** is called a *varicocele* and might relate to a low sperm count. An absent or *undescended testicle* (see chapter 3) might also be a clue to a hormonal imbalance.

The most important thing you can do to improve the genital examination is to drop your pants adequately. Some men will try to simply pull the penis through the zipper. Keeping in mind that half of the entire penis is located *inside* the body to begin with, the doctor may only be able to access as little as one-fourth of the penis if you just pull it out through the zipper. The testicles won't be accessible at all in that setting, so pull your pants and underwear down at least to the mid-thigh. Let the doctor do his work so you can move on to treatment.

THE RECTAL EXAMINATION

This is the biggie, the part of the urology appointment men dread the most. "I hate this," is the comment most often heard. Well, it ain't the high point of our day, either.

As unpleasant as many men think it is, the rectal examination should be performed annually on all men old enough to have significant disease that could be detected by doing so. That usually means rectal or **prostate** cancer, so the recommendations are usually to begin having a rectal examination after the age of fifty. Black men should begin five years earlier based on the increased risk of prostate cancer.

It's not rocket science, but there are a couple of things that help make the rectal examination more tolerable. First, you should try to get over any anxiety or embarrassment. Face it, the urologist sees essentially every patient's backside at some point, and yours isn't substantially different. None is exactly beautiful. The real reason to get over the anxiety is that nervousness makes the pelvic floor muscles tighten and lowers the pain threshold. That means the doctor has to push harder to get a gloved finger into the rectum, and more discomfort sensations will consequently be sent to the brain.

Some men complain about the amount of lubrication used on the gloved finger. Don't. Lubrication does more to lessen discomfort than anything else the doctor can do (except being gentle, which should be a given). The lubricating jelly is water-soluble, so washes or wipes off easily. Encourage him to use as much as needed.

Finally, your body position makes a big difference. Most men (and some doctors) don't know that the best position for a rectal examination is standing with the legs slightly apart. Leaning over an examining table with the knees slightly bent will allow your elbows to be placed at the *edge* of the examining table. This puts maximum bend into the waist, shortening the distance the doctor must reach inside to be able to check the prostate. The shorter distance means he pushes less—which is obviously in everyone's best interest. In obese men, this is the only way the urologist may be able to feel the entire prostate.

I GAVE AT THE OFFICE

The word *urologist* starts with *uro*, as in *urine*. That means that our specialty involves diseases that often exhibit findings in the urine. That also means that you shouldn't empty your bladder downstairs before coming into the office. You will be asked to give a specimen, so starting with an empty bladder means you will need to be given several paper cups full of water in order to refill the bladder. If you want to avoid the delay, save a donation until you check in.

Urosocopists were ancient physicians who made diagnoses by holding the patient's urine up to the light. They supposedly could see abnormalities that provided a view into the patient's constitution. So significant is the role of *uroscopy* in uromythology that the traditional logo of the *Journal of Urology* is a drawing of a urosocopist performing his craft. The *Journal of Urology* is the most prestigious journal in our field, but true to the mischievous nature of urologists, it was designated as "the official organ of the American Urological Association" for over fifty years. The journal retained its whimsical moniker until 1972, when some predictable ribbing by *Playboy* magazine made the editor relinquish the inside joke. The Europeans retain their sense of humor to this day and still call *European Urology* and the *Scandinavian Journal of Urology and Nephrology* "official organs."

No one today uses the appearance of urine held up to the light to make a diagnosis, but its appearance under the light of a microscope yields crucial information. Red or white blood cells indicate abnormalities of the urinary tract. Chemical tests for sugar indicate **diabetes**, a frequent cause of erectile dysfunction. Several other abnormalities can be easily detected through the urinalysis.

Blood tests are obtained in some patients by drawing blood through a small needle placed into a vein of the arm. The sample can be tested for testosterone to see if a deficiency is contributing to erectile dysfunction. **Prostate Specific Antigen (PSA)** screens for prostate cancer, as discussed in chapter 3. Chemical tests for diabetes, liver disease, kidney failure, and a number of other diseases might be performed if there is any suspicion.

Specialized tests to investigate the cause of erectile dysfunction are discussed in chapter 7. (The procedure for a prostate biopsy is discussed in chapter 3).

CYSTOSCOPY

The one specialized test performed in the urology office that deserves special attention is called **cystoscopy**. This is the placement of a small scope through the **urethra** into the urinary bladder. The scope is a relatively soft, flexible tube with *fiber optic* fibers running through it that allows the urologist to see the inside of the urethra, prostate, and *urinary bladder*. A gel containing *lidocaine* (the same anesthetic the dentist uses) is inserted into the urethra and bladder to decrease sensation. Then the cystoscope is inserted through the urethra in order to see the lower urinary tract. In our office, the patient can actually watch the same image that the urologist sees on a television screen. Photographs can be taken if anything abnormal is identified.

Cystoscopy is *not* part of the routine workup for erectile dysfunction, but it may be needed if abnormalities of the lower urinary tract are suspected. The most important use is to rule out cancer in someone who has blood in the urine, although stones, blockage, infections, incontinence, and other causes might indicate the need for cystoscopy as well.

The procedure is not usually painful, although most men describe mild discomfort or a "funny" sensation inside the penis. Cystoscopy is completed in minutes, and the urologist can immediately tell you the results of what he saw.

KEY POINTS

- Urologists are perhaps the most unusual group of medical and surgical specialists around.
- A doctor's appointment is for *your* good—not the doctor's. Therefore, make sure you communicate all your related history and symptoms to the physician.
- It is the doctor's responsibility to attempt to find out what your needs are from an appointment. Then he should determine the appropriate diagnostic evaluation and therapeutic options to assure these needs are met.
- It is the patient's responsibility to communicate all relevant information to the physician. If you ask the physician to give advice on the evaluation and management of your problem without making him aware of any related issues or history, you should expect inadequate

advice. This can lead to unsatisfactory, or occasionally dangerous, outcomes.

• The genitourinary and rectal examinations don't have to be intolerable. Work with your doctor.

Part Two
Treating Impotence
You Can Get Back in the Game

10 Relax—Maybe It's in Your Head

The penis does not obey the order of its master, who tries to erect
or shrink it at will. Instead, the penis erects freely while its master
is asleep. The penis must be said to have its own mind, by any
stretch of the imagination.

—Leonardo da Vinci

An erection may appear totally physical, but appearances can be
deceiving. Despite da Vinci's observation, the mind of the master
exerts considerable control over an erection. Specifically, it is the *nervous
(neurological) system* of the master that oversees the process. The brain is
the center of this. For this reason, we can observe that the most important
sex organ isn't between the legs—it's between the ears.

Unfortunately, these facts were long used to incorrectly assume erectile dysfunction was *all* "in the head." The father of all medicine, Hippocrates, attributed erectile dysfunction to a combination of overwork and
female unattractiveness. He believed that relaxing from work was one of
the few things that could remedy the situation.*

Not much changed in the following half-millennium. Until the very
late twentieth century, medical schools taught that 80 to 90 percent of men

---

*Which is also much easier and less risky than finding a more attractive partner.

were impotent due to mental causes. If men failed to improve, failure to resolve psychological issues was usually blamed.

In the last two decades, we have finally discovered that the opposite is true—80 to 90 percent of cases have physical, not mental, causes. However, although the greatest problems are physical, the mental aspects of erectile dysfunction can't be overlooked. Recall that in chapter 6 we learned that erectile dysfunction is rarely due to just one of the many factors involved in a normal erection. More often, a man begins having some slight decreased blood flow that he can compensate for. It is only when we add one or two other problems that he finally experiences erectile failure. The coup de grâce is often mental. When he begins fearing failure, the very stress of fearing so is the final blow. When he believes he can't get an erection, he will usually be right just by thinking so.

HOW DOES THE MIND AFFECT ERECTIONS?

If I convinced even the healthiest twenty-one-year-old male he had a condition that would prevent further erections, I would usually be right until he figured out I was lying. That may be an exaggeration for the twenty-one-year-old, but not for the man whose erections are beginning to take more effort. For many of these men, performance is fine as long as ideal conditions exist. However, when they start having difficulties, things can cascade out of hand quickly.

Ideal conditions for an erection involve both the physical and mental aspects. Physically, this means having normal blood flow into and out of the penis, as well as normal hormones and generally decent health. Mentally, it's more complex. There must be at least some combination of stimulation and arousal, which paradoxically requires at least some relaxation as well. This also has to be in an environment where he is not too anxious or depressed. He can't be impaired by medications, including alcohol, tobacco, or illicit drugs. Finally, the five senses continually affect the mental landscape.

In other words, there are multiple ways for things to fall apart mentally.

THE FIVE SENSES: SETTING THE STAGE FOR SUCCESS

As a sensory organ, the penis is limited to touch alone among the five senses. It has no sense of sight, sound, smell, or taste. If the penis were the only male body part with a role in sex, this would be the end of the story. However, the remaining senses play a major role above the waist.

Sight is the source of about 90 percent of our sensory input. Regarding sexual activity, the most obvious role of sight is in perception of a partner's attractiveness. Hippocrates put a lot of credibility on this, but many other visual factors come into play. Some people are more comfortable sexually in darker places. This might be related to their own taboos involving sex, or they may be uncomfortable with the physical appearance of their own or their partners' bodies. The dark can hide many inadequacies, physical or mental. Others find that having enough light to see well leads to improved stimulation. Candlelight presents a mood some people find arousing, while others are excited more in colored or other artificial light. Whichever lighting intensity and scheme you find helpful, it is important to recognize its impact on both partners.

Sound may help some people be either more comfortable or more stimulated. Many people find music helps set the mood, distracting them from the pressure total silence creates. Obviously, the sounds of a partner may be stimulating or distracting. Even worse, the sounds of the kids down the hall, a mother-in-law in the next room, the neighbors arguing, or the answering machine recording the boss's voice can ruin an otherwise hopeful attempt.

Smell (which is interrelated with *taste*) is the most overlooked sensation. Taste usually doesn't play a role of great importance, but fresh breath on both ends of a kiss is worth the three cents or so for the toothpaste. The part of the brain that senses smell is intimately connected to the *limbic system*, the place our strongest emotions are held. The limbic system is the most primitive part of the brain, so emotions held here can be primal in nature. Since sex is such an emotional experience, an integration of smells can greatly influence enjoyment, success, and how memories preserve the occasion. Remember the perfume your partner wore the first time you held each other close? It would be a much more arousing aroma than would be the smell of athletic socks hanging off the bedpost. A shower or bath before going to bed isn't a bad idea if you had a long, hot, sweaty day; your partner's response to your scent will make her more likely to be interested as well.

Pheromones are chemical substances that use the sense of smell to send signals between animals. The most striking example involves a female dog in heat, arousing male dogs for miles around with the fragrance. The role of pheromones in humans is less clear. It has been hypothesized that women produce pheromones during the portion of their menstrual cycle when fertilization is possible. Some researchers believe this uses the sense of smell to facilitate sexual activity in humans.

The role of *touch* in sexual experience is obvious, but there are other ways touch matters. Clean, fresh sheets take away the chance you will notice them instead of each other. Dry skin won't be nearly as well received as clean skin moistened with even a simple moisturizer.

In summary, a culmination of the input of all five senses lays the groundwork upon which the sexual experience will be based.

THE MIND: IT'S A TERRIBLE THING TO WASTE ON SEX

> Anxiety is the first time a man can't get it up twice.
> Panic is the second time he can't get it up once.
>
> —Anonymous

The first time a man suffers erectile dysfunction, it's alarming. The second may create a crisis—at least in his mind. He may become obsessed with achieving an erection. You might guess this doesn't lay the groundwork for a successful quick recovery. Each time anxiety increases, success is one step further away. To paraphrase Franklin Delano Roosevelt, the fear itself may become worse than the underlying problem.

This phenomenon is called **performance anxiety**. Like all other forms of anxiety, it is only partially mental. Mentally, the person feels he can't perform. This feeling of helplessness is enough of a problem. Unfortunately, a worse problem may be due to the physical chemicals the body releases during such times. These chemicals (mainly *adrenalin*) are responsible for the feelings of anxiety we all recognize: chest tightening, heart racing, trembling, shaking, nausea, etc. Obviously, anyone experiencing these symptoms may be a little less prone to have an erection. Not so obvious is the effect these chemicals have on the blood vessels going to the penis. These substances are **vasoconstrictors**, the agents that constrict or close vessels down. If these blood vessels are already limited in their ability to carry enough blood for an erection, they sure won't be helped by further narrowing from these chemicals. This is similar to what happens during smoking.

Studies have shown that simply having increased levels of adrenalin can make laboratory animals unable to have erections. Likewise, men with performance anxiety will kill any hope for an erection if these chemicals are allowed to storm their systems. These chemicals in excess can harm more than an erection. They can lead to high blood pressure, heart disease, and stroke. Not a good way to deal with the problem.

EXAMPLES OF PERFORMANCE ANXIETY

> Sudden fear, or anything which fixes our attention strongly and all at once, makes this member quickly subside, though it were ever so fully erect.
> —Robert Whytt, *An Essay on the Vital and Other Involuntary Motions of Animals*, 1751

Lenny took his erections for granted. Whenever he went to bed, they were as reliable as his alarm clock. One Saturday night after a long evening on the town with his wife, Anne, he finished off a final beer and headed upstairs for their Saturday night routine. Anne was asleep by the time he got there. She was willing to wake up and be receptive, but only after some cajoling. Amid the beers, his exhaustion, and Anne's sleepiness, he wasn't very stimulated. The harder he tried, the more upset he got. He finally gave up and fell asleep unsatisfied.

The following day Lenny pondered the events. "What is wrong with me?" he wondered. That night he was committed to proving to Anne that he was as virile as ever. When the erection wasn't already standing out as he crawled in bed, he panicked. Several ill-fated attempts were made to achieve an erection before both of them rolled over in disappointment. Neither of them even tried to touch each other the following night.

The most common example of performance anxiety is among men who have always had easy erections, but then experience their first brush with impotence. This might be at a time when they were tired or stressed, or maybe after drinking more than usual. Maybe the erection took more effort to achieve during a sexual encounter when the partner wasn't encouraging. This brush with inadequacy then fosters seeds of doubt that are in mind the next time the opportunity arises. If he thinks—or worries—about it too much, the stage is set for failure. Lenny was in this situation.

This pattern is called a **vicious cycle**. This means that two problems propagate each other. In this situation, a momentary difficulty is usually the instigating step. However, once this occurs, the panic makes it even more difficult to achieve an erection. Then, the next time the man has an even greater difficulty achieving an erection, leading to even more panic. And so it goes . . .

Men in this situation often describe themselves having something like an out-of-body experience. As foreplay begins, many envision it in the third person as if they can picture themselves about to have problems. They foresee the penis going soft, at which point it's almost inevitable that it really will do so. This occurrence has been called **spectatoring**.

This is the time to nip the problem in the bud. As the saying goes, just getting back up on the pony is usually the best cure. Once convinced everything still works the same, most men won't have any further problems. Unfortunately, many men don't get back up on the pony. Instead, they worry, fret, and drive themselves into a psychological corner. Panic sets in. If the pattern is left untouched, recovery becomes more difficult with each subsequent failure. The vicious cycle is spinning its ugly wheels—a runaway train at this point.

The partner plays a major role at this juncture. If she is supportive and gently tries to reassure him everything is all right, there's a good chance it will be. This is easier said than done. More often, those same seeds of doubt or anxiety are planted in her mind as well. In fact, they may be worse for her, since she has to deal not only with her interpretation of what's going on, but also has to try to figure out what's going on in his mind as well. That's a lot to deal with.

Sometimes, her doubts take on a life of their own. She may wonder if he doesn't find her attractive anymore. Even worse, she may question if he still loves her or suspect he is having an affair. That might stoke her anxiety a little bit! Attacking the mental aspects will be critical to long-term success. Without doing so, most couples will continue to have sexual problems for a long time.

One of the first questions I ask men involves whether either of these is true. If there are marital difficulties, these need to be worked out before going much further. Otherwise, we're only trying to patch up a sinking ship.

If he is truly having an affair and erections are no problem with the other partner, we have a real problem. I first point out I'm not a marital counselor, and that he probably needs one. This is a classic situation where the mental aspects of sex are controlling the situation. There is no easy answer, but he needs to sort things out in the bedroom quickly, or his life may spiral downwards quickly. His problems may move from the bedroom to the courtroom (or the boardroom if things are happening at work or affecting his work).

If it's an attraction issue, counseling may be needed to deal with the fact she's not still twenty-one and shaped like a cheerleader. Of course, he's not necessarily the shining knight he was on their first date, but as they go through life together, hopefully they remain on somewhat equal planes so things stay fair. It seems that we are biologically programmed to find appropriate partners appealing. Studies show that couples tend to possess somewhat similar levels of attractiveness.

I believe this tendency also includes an adaptive mechanism for aging. Therefore, we usually don't find middle-aged women attractive when we're teens; however, by the time we're graying ourselves, women of that age are as attractive to us as teenagers were when we were adolescents.

HOW COULD I POSSIBLY RELAX?

If a woman's hand, which is the best of all remedies, is not good enough to cure the flabbiness of a man's penis, the other remedies will do little.

—N. Vennette, *Conjugal Love*

It's easy to tell these men to relax, but obviously, relaxation is not usually their strong suit. They must take it a little further. "Getting it off your chest" can work wonders, especially if a couple is capable of talking openly about such issues. Most are not—at least not well.

For these couples, counseling might be wise. Yes, it sounds like "Dear Abby," but counseling can work wonders for those who need a neutral ground. Counseling should usually be done by someone who specializes in sexual issues. Your counselor for nonsexual issues may not be comfortable talking about such intimate details. If you are considering using their services for erectile dysfunction, you should ask for a frank opinion from them on whether they are comfortable with taking on this part of your counseling. Even more important is to avoid asking people who will be judgmental to counsel you for sexual issues. Clergymen may be able to counsel the flock on a number of matters, but few are prepared to really take an open-minded approach to your sex life. Asking such persons to provide sexual counseling is not only unlikely to work, but also risks damage to your relationship with them.

Masters and Johnson set the tone for sex therapy with their ground-breaking work in the middle of the twentieth century. Their book, *Human Sexual Response*,[1] was the first (and still most complete) work to quantify the subject of its title. Their controversial work involving direct observation of people having sex led to their form of sex therapy, sensate focus. Sensate focus is an intensive regimen designed to help men (or women) with desire/arousal difficulties. Couples are instructed to begin slowly with nonsexual contact (rubbing necks, backs, arms, etc.) in order to allow relaxation and release of inhibitions. They are then to progress slowly to increasing levels of intimacy, and are allowed genital contact only after a prolonged period (several sessions) of progress. Eventually, the partners are allowed to initiate genital contact without intercourse, including mutual masturbation and **ejaculation** if desired. Only after achieving total relaxation are they supposed to attempt intercourse. It at that time, either partner is not ready, they are instructed to back off to contact that is perceived as being less stressful or anxiety-provoking.

Success is sometimes acknowledged when both partners reach levels of arousal that they disregard instructions to hold back. When they both say "to hell with it" and progress to intercourse, this may be the signal that further therapy is no longer needed.

Sensate focus can be a curative option for many couples with psychological issues such as performance anxiety or ejaculatory disorders, but the work required dissuades many of those who would benefit from it.

MANAGING DIFFICULT CASES OF PERFORMANCE ANXIETY

To help these men move forward, oral medications are often prescribed even though the problem is "between the ears." The reason is twofold. First, the increased ease of obtaining an erection while taking the medication makes continued failures less likely. Perhaps more importantly, the confidence of knowing the medication is on board goes a long way toward overcoming the performance anxiety—"confidence in a little blue pill," as one patient described it. After couples experience success, the medications can usually be weaned quickly as the pharmacological and psychological boost becomes unnecessary.

SOME THINGS THAT DON'T WORK

> With her hand, she began to stroke that part of me which by now was cold as ice, shriveled with a thousand deaths.
> —Gaius Petronius (27–66 c.e.)

Unfortunately, men sometimes take matters into their own hands in counter-productive ways. A long-established curative attempt was infidelity, often with prostitutes or others perceived to be "a sure thing." Don't do this.* Success in this situation is no more proof of the ability to get an erection and perform than is masturbation. Therefore, proving the ability to get erect doesn't solve the problem. It doesn't mean you can get an erection when and where you need—it just means you can get an erection, period. However, difficulties may still occur in the same situation where problems were originally noted. Therefore, the erection may still fail in the same old situation.

The ability to have an erection can be determined just as easily by looking in your shorts upon waking in the morning or by using the "postage stamp test" as outlined in chapter 7. That may instill confidence, but the erection still has to work when the pressure is on with a partner.

Instead, infidelity (especially with a prostitute) risks guilt feelings at best and a divorce at worst, with some really nasty diseases in between. Your goal is to achieve an erection in a specific setting. Don't try to prove your flying skills in a boat. What most men need is a caring, understanding partner to support them in a difficult situation. Caring and understanding aren't typically included in a prostitute's fee.

Withholding sex from the female partner is foolhardy. The idea is this: "If I don't approach her for some prolonged time, she will become ravenous and will aggressively pursue me." Yeah, right. In reality, she may be relieved that his frustrated attempts have stopped and erroneously conclude he is no longer interested. She may next draw the reasonable conclusion their sex life has ended. The man may become more desperate when she doesn't respond voraciously as he planned, which may place even more stress in the situation. Either way, it's not going to work.

---

*Recall King David's ill-fated attempt with Abishag.

Some couples find pornographic films or other materials arousing, but only if both members are equally comfortable with these things. Otherwise, it is likely to increase stress between the two. The same can be said for "sex toys" and other erotica. A couple believing these tools would be helpful should probably be in a counseling situation, as inevitably there will be some disparity in their interests.

Spanish fly, the favorite snack of history's most famous pervert, the Marquis de Sade, has been used to improve erections for centuries. Made from the ground wings of the bug otherwise known as the *blister beetle*, there is no scientific evidence it works as noted earlier. There is plenty of proof it causes abdominal pain, seizures, rectal bleeding, erosion of mucosal surfaces (the lining of the organs), and internal bleeding. Deaths can occur from these side effects. In fact, the only effective medical use of the active ingredient in Spanish fly is for wart removal: it melts them away. Pretty stimulating.

NEW PARTNER SYNDROME

> For once a man has been capable with a certain woman, he will
> never be incapable with her again unless out of real impotence
> —Michel de Montaigne, 1580

Single life was hard on Bob. The marriage to his high school sweetheart fell apart after five years. He had been with only a couple of previous sexual partners, so the whole dating game was uncomfortable for him.

He ran into Kim, a girl he'd always had a crush on during college. She was attractive, intelligent, and the youngest daughter of a local politician. Her own marriage had ended two years earlier, but no subsequent suitor had caught her attention for long. They agreed to meet for dinner.

After six hours of comfortable conversation, they both found more in common than either would have suspected. Several more dates followed, and it became clear to each of them that this was promising. Bob looked forward to the future for the first time in several years. He worshiped everything about her and felt like the luckiest man in the world that she seemed to share his affection. After only a few dates, their discussions became more pointed, wandering to such issues as children and future plans. Unspoken, they both knew that marriage was a reasonable direction this relationship was heading.

After dinner at Kim's apartment, the moment they both knew was coming arrived. They ended up in the bedroom to consummate the relationship. Things started out great, but when the sheets were turned down, so was Bob. Twenty months after his last sexual experience, he became panic-stricken. He made up an excuse that he felt ill and left in a hurry.

Kim was a little embarrassed but brought him dinner the next evening. He clearly felt physically well. They talked about their near-encounter, and they agreed they both wanted a sexual relationship to be part of what they agreed was possibly to become a marital relationship. Soon, they were heading to Bob's bedroom to close the deal.

Disaster struck. Stepping across the threshold, Bob started fearing a repeat performance. He was right. He couldn't even undress for fear of embarrassment. Kim tried to get him to talk about it, but he had nothing else to say.

Each lay awake in separate beds later that evening. Bob was convinced that he was unworthy of such a woman and that his erection was just one example of this. Kim was convinced he didn't find her attractive and obviously didn't care for her in the way she had believed only twenty-four hours earlier. It was a sleepless night in their neighborhood.

The second type of performance anxiety often involves the most dramatic cases—the new partner syndrome. This may be someone who has just gotten out of a bad marriage, or someone whose wife left him against his wishes. Maybe his wife of many years died. Sometimes it is just a man who waited until later than typical in life to become sexually active (usually due to waiting until marriage for moral or religious reasons).

Some of these men have dated around and often had no problem with one-night stands. However, when they are in it for serious rather than just for fun, the pressure begins. Finally in a serious relationship, they find themselves suddenly in a high-pressure situation they weren't prepared for. They develop incapacitating performance anxiety that can be difficult to overcome.

The very nature of these men being on the dating market for the first time in years is a setup for difficulties. They have often had little or no sexual activity during the waning years of a previous relationship. In fact, sexual issues may have been a major part of their marital difficulties. After all, it was a marriage on the rocks. On the other hand, in the situation of a widower, his deceased wife may have been ill for some time, making sexual activity unlikely as well.

There are many varied reasons men have this experience. Many may be dealing with issues left over from a previous relationship. They may be ambivalent about becoming involved with a new partner or may feel guilty about sexual activity outside a previously monogamous relationship. Widowers may feel unfaithful to the deceased partner.

Like Bob, these men are almost universally nice guys. Jerks don't worry like that, so rarely will this be an issue for them. These men are often well educated or professionals. They have frequently found "the one," the woman they believe holds the key to their future happiness. Often, she is someone they suspect is above their own level—"too good for me." This common feeling may be based on either attractiveness or social stature.

Bob and Kim finally got back together a week later when she called to confront him. "I really thought you loved me. I know I loved you."

Bob was floored. He had spent the entire week feeling unworthy of the one woman of his dreams. They acknowledged their mutual adoration and were together in Kim's apartment within the hour, with the expressed intent to make it work this time. The stakes were high and the pressure was on. Kim tried everything she knew to arouse him, but each time he got an erection, he started fearing it would go away. It did go away every time they tried to have intercourse, until he finally decided to go away as well.

Performance anxiety combined with these feelings of unworthiness is particularly debilitating. They believe that if they can't perform sexually, their chance of holding onto her is nil. They try harder and harder. Often, there is a definite "date" they are gearing up for, and they are panicked that they won't be able to perform for such a big curtain call. This is a recipe for disaster.

The first thing these men must do is to take the pressure off. Who could perform under the pressure of knowing that failure to have an erection will mean losing the "love of my life"? Although any of the temporary treatments for erectile dysfunction may help get them through the night, their fear of failure must abate if they are to have any chance of long-term success.

This involves an open dialogue between the partners. My approach has been to advise a man suffering from this problem that, if she is the "right one," she will understand his hopes and fears and work supportively with him. If she won't, he should question whether she is right for him in the long term anyway. In situations where the woman wouldn't stick by her man, her departure has always been in his best interest. I can't remember a time in which he didn't deserve better.

Success still comes only by getting "back up on the horse." Once he can relax enough to perform satisfactorily a couple times, the problem usually goes away. Then it becomes just a good story they can laugh about later in the relationship. As you might guess, this is far easier said than done, and a large number of these couples break up. This is often a shame, since it's the fact that he's so committed to making it work that starts the vicious circle.

Bob came to the office in a panic. "I'm going to lose her if I can't keep an erection." It didn't take much discussion to get to the bottom of this one. He readily acknowledged, on direct questioning, that she was the woman of his dreams. He felt she was above him both physically and socially. He believed his lifetime of happiness hung in the balance, with his performance standing between success and failure.

On Kim's end, the only explanation she could deduce was that he wasn't attracted to her. Otherwise, how could he not be aroused by her advances?

The assistance of medication, combined with my reassurance that he had normal anatomy and that his testosterone blood test was normal, allowed Bob to finally relax enough to make love to Kim successfully. Success only came when they understood each other fully. He was able to confess his total commitment to her. He explained the pressure he felt and how the fear of losing her was so overwhelming. Once she understood that his problem was desiring her too much—not the opposite—she was able to confidently and patiently work with him. The pressure was lessened, so things finally fell into place. After a second successful encounter the following night, they never looked back. The last two tablets were never used.

SEXUAL IDENTITY: WE ALL HAVE OUR OWN VIEWPOINT OF SEX

Phil was raised in a traditional Catholic nuclear family. Sex was not discussed openly or otherwise. Phil had never believed his parents had been sexually active outside the fertilization of their four children. Despite a rigid upbringing, all the children were straight-laced, with two of the sisters becoming nuns and the other becoming a kindergarten teacher.

When Phil finally went to college, he quickly began to sow his oats, experiencing several sexual relationships. He never became close enough with any of these college girlfriends to consider marriage until he met

Michelle his senior year. She was from a public high school in his home-town, and although he had noticed her a couple times during high school, they had never actually met. When they began dating, it was clear they were compatible and both wanted to settle in their hometown. Easily set-ting religious differences aside, they began to discuss marriage after only a few weeks.

Phil never tried to take the physical aspect of their relationship beyond heavy petting until Michelle made it clear that more was not only accept-able, but also desired. It was clear she was as sexually experienced as he was when they finally slept together. On the first few occasions, things went fine. Then he began to think. Although he had no problems with sexual activity with any previous partner, Phil was uncomfortable with Michelle's open attitude toward sex. He had an image in his mind of a marital partner mirroring his own mother—chaste and proper, a traditional wife and mother dedicated mainly to raising children. Michelle fit the "proper" role and was clearly interested in being a homemaker, but her sexual openness made Bill question her entire being. Did this mean she wasn't the chaste and proper mother he desired for his own children? Phil began to seriously question whether this meant she was not the person he wanted to marry.

This couple was clearly in love and well suited to each other, but Phil was having a personal crisis trying to sort out which type of girl he should date versus which type he should marry. He didn't think one girl could be both. On his first visit, he came alone. This allowed him to discuss openly how much he cared for her. My first suspicion was the new partner syn-drome, but his early success with Michelle made it clear that such a simple answer wasn't adequate.

When Michelle accompanied him on the second visit, it was obvious why he would want to marry her. She was well suited to him in every vis-ible way, pleasant, and supportive. Although by no means dowdy, it was easy to imagine her assuming a maternal role. So, what could be the problem?

They agreed to counseling after it became clear Phil's discomfort regarding Michelle's sexuality was standing in the way. After just a few sessions, Bill's conflicting feelings about sex—"it's okay for fun, but good girls don't enjoy it"—were brought out in the open. It took a while for him to resolve this conflict, which was a throwback to his own childhood, but the couple committed to each other. The last time I saw them, marriage plans were in the works. Both agreed their sex life had never been better.

❂   ❂   ❂

Each of us has a *sexual identity* that goes well beyond sexual orientation. It involves how we view sex and what we feel is normal and acceptable sexual behavior. This begins forming early in life, often by observing small glimpses of our parents' interactions. Unfortunately, these glimpses offer only a minimal view of normal sexual interactions. We may see healthy parental interactions, like a warm embrace in front of the fireplace. On the other hand, we may hear groans through the wall that certainly won't send reassuring signals about healthy sexual interactions when heard by a small child. Some children find items in their parents' bedroom that stoke curiosity and often revulsion. With only partial information, the message often ends up being, "sex is dirty—save it for someone you love."

We may also get sexual information from direct discussion with parents. Open discussion starting early in life is best, but many families aren't able to achieve this in a healthy manner. Often, this is part of a longstanding cycle—the grandparents couldn't deal well with such matters, so the parents of subsequent generations aren't prepared either. Phil's parents never spoke of sex or showed signs that sex was acceptable for anything but procreation. This left Phil to define his own sexual identity with inadequate information.

Understanding one's sexual identity is never straightforward. Understanding that of one's partner is even harder. When ideology is not too different between the partners, simply talking about things openly is adequate. This might involve minor disagreements about the frequency, location, or spontaneity of intercourse.

Some couples will have completely different views of what is acceptable or desired. When major differences exist, counseling is almost always required to make much progress. Difficulties may arise regarding use of sex paraphernalia, sexual positions, oral sex, etc. Especially difficult would be differences in how each views infidelity. There is no circumstance where infidelity helps a relationship, and this may in fact be the most divisive sexual issue. This one usually won't (or maybe shouldn't) be fixed unless the offending partner does a permanent U-turn.

JOHN AND CAROL: EVOLVING SEXUAL IDENTITIES

Through twelve years of marriage, John and Carol were both satisfied with intercourse almost nightly. When Carol went through menopause, she maintained interest in sex but often experienced vaginal dryness and discomfort following more than one or two days of intercourse in a row. She assumed John would understand her changing body based on their discussion one day after her routine gynecological appointment. The gynecologist had even prescribed vaginal estrogen cream for the symptoms. John never complained about the decreased frequency, which was by that time about twice a week.

While on vacation they tried to regain their daily routine. After one occasion in which Carol actually winced in pain during penetration, John couldn't maintain an erection. After that, there was no intercourse for over two weeks. He came to my office sullen and quiet, complaining of erectile dysfunction.

After just a few questions, it became clear John wasn't impotent at all. He continued to have normal erections most mornings and had masturbated only the day before. Instead, it was obvious that he had become threatened by Carol's rather sudden decrease in **libido** and comfort with intercourse. He couldn't keep an erection because he feared it would cause the same reaction in Carol again.

Several issues are evident in John and Carol's story. Most significant is John's sudden anxiety over a single episode when things didn't go according to plan. Had he been able to relax and let things go back to normal as soon as Carol's physical discomfort abated, I would have never met them. Typically, he overreacted and things spiraled out of hand.

Not as obvious is the role their changing sexual identities played. John had difficulty accepting two normal parts of aging—Carol's menopause, and their natural decrease in intercourse frequency. John's sexual view called for daily intercourse. Carol's sexual view accepted this frequency, but didn't demand it, so when she had physical reasons to slow down she did so without hesitation. John's interpretation was rejection.

Fortunately, once they both were able to communicate their viewpoints clearly, it became acceptable to both to have intercourse one or two times a week. They found that with their decreased frequency, they actually began looking forward to intercourse more and enjoyed their sex lives more than previously. They agreed to prioritize quality over quantity, leaving both more satisfied not only sexually, but with the relationship as well.

John and Carol's story demonstrates how sexual identity changes throughout our lifetimes. For teenagers, it revolves around the questions, "How far and with whom?" For young adults it may mean intercourse regularly, decreasing with age to the point it is scheduled or planned around the calendar. For the elderly, it may become an anniversary event or go by the wayside completely. The important thing is to understand your own view and to try to meld that as closely as feasible to your partner's.

What if sexual views are too divergent? This is a problem. Most commonly, men desire intercourse on a more frequent and more adventuresome basis than women, but not always. Most couples can find a happy medium if motivated to work with each other. The more interested partner may accept the compromise, while the less interested partner may acquiesce in order to find a middle ground. If an acceptable compromise is not reached, masturbation provides a release for some, while others take the hazardous approach of infidelity or sex with prostitutes. Whatever it takes, including counseling if needed, don't let things spiral to this point.

KEY POINTS

- The most important sex organ isn't between the legs—it's between the ears.
- If a man believes he can't get an erection, he is usually right. One of the first steps is making him believe.
- Performance anxiety blocks the ability to achieve an erection, both mentally and physically.
- The new partner syndrome is often due to a man's feeling unworthy of his new mate.
- Counseling is helpful to couples dealing with erectile dysfunction that is primarily psychogenic in nature. The most intense form, sensate focus, is reserved for couples highly motivated to permanently dispense with severe psychological inhibitions.
- All persons have a unique sexual identity. Understanding this viewpoint and matching it with the viewpoint of a partner is the most likely recipe for success.

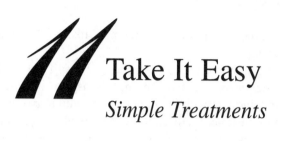

Take It Easy

Simple Treatments

The mystery of sex presents itself to the young, not as a scientific problem to be solved, but as a romantic emotion to be accounted for. The only result of the current endeavor to explain its phenomena by seeking parallels in botany is to make botany obscene.
—H. L. Mencken, 1919

*P*rescription medications and surgery aren't the answer for all men concerned with erectile dysfunction. Sometimes a little boost is all that is needed. This most often takes the form of devices designed to augment an erection. Alternatively, complementary medical treatments are popular, although evidence of their effectiveness is lacking.

VACUUM CONSTRICTION DEVICES (VCDs)

Ben and Jane, married for forty-eight years, had intercourse almost every Saturday night. Smoking finally caught up with Ben, making his erections become unreliable. He wasn't truly impotent, but many times an adequate erection at the beginning of intercourse became barely sufficient following penetration. Jane was cooperative but not overly motivated to continue the routine.

Although an ideal candidate for oral therapy, Ben despised anything modern or medical. The idea of taking a pill seemed objectionable to him, so he struggled with the problem until he became more likely to fail than succeed on any given attempt.

At that point, he was finally willing to talk about it. He still refused to take medications, but after a long and frustrating discussion, he finally agreed to schedule an appointment with the impotence coordinator at least to consider options. He immediately refused to even think about anything invasive but was intrigued by a demonstration of a **vacuum constriction device (VCD)**.

One attempt was convincing. Without anything he considered *medical*, the VCD provided an erection Ben could be proud, and confident, of. Saturday evenings were successful once again.

Vacuum constriction devices are cylinders designed to create a vacuum around the penis. Negative pressure inside the cylinders causes blood to flow into the **corpora cavernosae**. When the penis becomes full enough to become erect, a band is allowed to gently constrict around the base of the penis so the pressure remains long enough for intercourse (see Fig. 4)

Patent holder Otto Lederer is generally credited with inventing vacuum devices, but he was not even close. Dr. John King built his first one in 1874 using a concept actually envisioned at the University of Leiden over a century earlier. Interestingly, this was the same location where Dr. Patrick Walsh joined with Dr. Pieter Donker in 1981 to finally identify where the nerves to the penis were located, a significant discovery that finally allowed surgeons to perform **radical prostatectomy** (removal of the prostate) without making men impotent (see chapter 2).

Researchers at the University of Leiden had observed that the lungs naturally fill passively by the vacuum created during chest wall expansion. They subsequently found that a balloon inside a vacuum jar filled with air as a vacuum was created within the jar. This prototype became the model for using negative pressure (a vacuum) to fill an object.

This concept is now used to expand the balloon known as the penis using a similar technique. Dr. Lederer received U.S. patent number 1,225,341 in 1917 when he proved a vacuum device could fill the penis. His invention went unappreciated for decades until Geddings Osbon introduced the first commercial device in 1974. He reputedly wasn't satisfied with being told erectile dysfunction was in his head, so had made his own VCD. With FDA approval eight years later, he had the first successful nonsurgical treatment option for erectile dysfunction. The first model, called the Youth Equivalent Device, required mouth suction on its tubing. The hand pumps

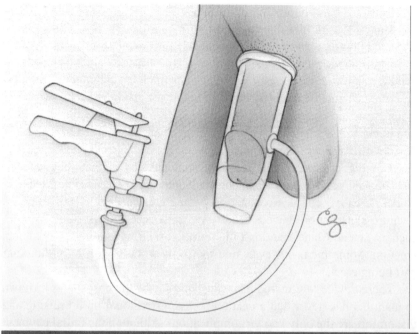

Fig. 4. Vacuum contriction device (VCD). A hand pump creates a vacuum in this example, whereas other versions utilize an electric pump.

and electric suctions that followed were more palatable and commercially successful.

The first VCDs were controversial at best. Many physicians suspected they were gimmicks. The U.S. Postal Service actually banned their shipment under their interpretation the devices were "pornographic." Dr. Osbon's device required a prescription until the FDA in 1997 suspended this requirement. His and similar devices are now readily available to anyone wanting a noninvasive, nonprescription treatment for erectile dysfunction.

THE PENIS IN A VACUUM

The device is typically composed of a hollow plastic cylinder large enough to fit easily over the penis. This cylinder is seated against the body wall, using lubricating gel to create an airtight seal. A vacuum is created by either an electric or hand pump. When sufficient negative pressure is generated, the penis fills with blood just as it does in a normal erection. Clear plastic housing allows easy visual confirmation that the erection is adequate.

After the vacuum fills the penis, an elastic band is then slipped off the cylinder onto the penile shaft where it exits the body. This keeps the portion of penis outside the body erect by holding in the blood. The portion of penis inside the body becomes soft immediately, but usually this outer portion being full is adequate. Most men have an adequate erection with these devices after proper instruction.

The biggest complaint about vacuum devices is that they are too "mechanical" and reduce spontaneity. It may not be spontaneous, but it works. Creative couples can actually integrate the device into foreplay. Vacuum constriction devices tend to be most accepted by stable couples such as Ben and Jane that don't mind the extra effort required to obtain an erection. Some men, however, find the penis wobbly with only the outer part being erect.

These devices are incredibly safe. This may be the only therapy known to man that has never had a death reported. Occasional mild bruising and discomfort are the only known complications. Although the initial payment may be a few hundred dollars, they are virtually indestructible and may last a lifetime. Most insurance plans and Medicare cover part or all of the cost.

Obese men comprise the one group of men that usually won't be satisfied with VCDs. The vacuum requires that the cylinder be seated securely against the body wall. Therefore, a large belly will make this difficult.

Improper seating of the device against the body wall can make it difficult to produce the vacuum. At best, this means not enough suction is produced, so the penis never gets erect. At worst, any loose body parts nearby can be drawn inside. There aren't too many structures near the penis you'd want to be accidentally pulled in, so men master the process quickly. Finally, some couples report a coolness to the penis that is based on the relatively low level of continued blood flow through the organ while the **constriction ring** is in place.

The type of pump doesn't make much difference. The electric (battery operated) pump is a little easier to use, but isn't necessarily more effective. The hand pump works just as well and costs less. As long as an adequate vacuum is created, whether electrically or manually, the device should work.

A VCD IN YOUR VCR

The most important, and most overlooked, factor in determining the success of a VCD is education. It is clear that men who are trained properly in the urologist's office usually have success. Men who obtain the device out of a catalog, over the Internet, or in a drugstore rarely achieve satisfying results. The reason is that they must be shown how to create and keep an adequate vacuum long enough to place the constriction ring. Without instruction, most won't achieve success.

Therefore, success rates are hard to interpret, but most men who buy one are happy with the devices when properly trained and motivated. At my clinic, we usually have our **impotence coordinator** teach the technique. The Osbon Corporation (now part of the Timm Corporation of Eden Prairie, Minnesota), as well as some of the other reliable manufacturers, will actually come to the physician's office to meet and teach patients as well, so there is no good reason not to be properly instructed in their use.

Some cheap knockoff VCDs are sold with poorly written instructions that may only frustrate the customers. Although most VCDs come with a VCR demonstration tape, it is no substitute for proper training in person. In fact, some VCD VCR tapes are barely more than soft porn, so don't count on them to teach the technique properly.

RINGING TRUE

"It just goes back down as soon as I get inside my wife," Charles lamented. His erection was early to rise, but early to fall. The problem had been progressively worsening for two or three years, culminating with mutual frustration that led them to quit trying. At fifty-six, this wasn't an acceptable option to either Charles or Beth, so he asked for help.

An initial attempt using Viagra slowed down the decline in his erection, but still didn't allow Charles to keep an erection of sufficient duration. It was clear that Charles suffered from **venous insufficiency**—incompetent valves in the veins exiting the penis that allowed the blood to flow out too quickly. I recommended he try a constriction ring in order to slow down the outflow. He tried several different types of constriction rings, settling on the **Actis ring** (see Fig. 5). As soon as he achieved a complete erection, he placed the ring around the base of his penis and secured it just tightly enough to impede outflow. During penetration, neither he nor his wife

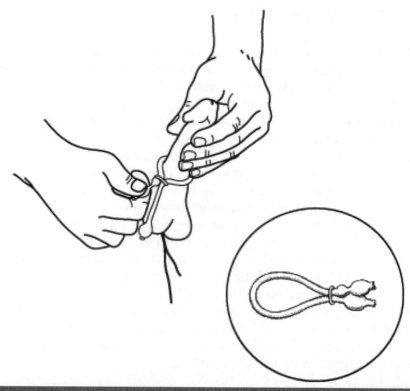

Fig. 5. Actis constriction ring secured around base of penis.
(Illustration courtesy of Vivus Corporation, Mountain View, California).

could feel the ring in place. Both were satisfied with the erection and its duration thereafter.

Rings placed tightly around the base of the penis have been used for centuries to sustain an erection. In Medieval times these were known by their distasteful nickname, *cock rings*, and were made with leather, metals, or animal horns. Similar devices are available currently that are more humane and more effective. They can be used alone or in combination with vacuum devices.

The mechanism of action for constriction rings is to impede blood flow out of the corporal bodies. For men with **venous insufficiency** (see chapter 6), these rings compensate for the inadequate venous valves and keep the tire fully inflated until intercourse is complete. For many men simply noticing a slight decrease in erections, this impedance may make enough difference to be all that some will require.

THE RINGS

The most common constriction rings are made by the Osbon Corporation, the original developer and leading manufacturer of **VCDs**. Their rings are a thick, practically indestructible rubber with a large central circle and smaller handles on either side. They are designed to fit on a VCD but also do well as constriction rings on their own. Their rubber is slightly sticky, so they can pull at skin or hair if not used carefully.

The Vivus Corporation sells a constriction ring that some men find easier to use. Their Actis ring is designed like a tourniquet. It is made of a softer latex, so it's less likely to pull skin or hair. This softer latex may not be as durable, but it is reusable for at least six months. More flexible and more comfortable for most men, it will expand to a larger diameter in order to slip on more easily. It is designed to be used with their MUSE product (a medical pellet inserted into the urethra as described in chapter 13) but is valuable for any man desiring restriction of blood flow out of the penis.

THE WRONG (W)RING!

Sometimes men make their own constriction rings. Disaster is likely. When metal or other nonexpandable materials are used, they can get stuck. The penis beyond the ring expands (that's the idea), so it becomes larger than the hole it sticks through. Therefore, it can't be pulled back out. The longer it stays in the ring, the more it expands. This is yet another **vicious cycle**— one that will inevitably end up as a most embarrassing trip to the emergency room.

Some of the most fascinating emergency room visits involve men who have creatively made their own constriction rings. Some of the most remarkable include metal pipe rings, barbell weights, wedding rings, and various pieces of machinery. Some men put their own bolts inside large threaded nuts. The hardest I've seen was a wood-splitting maul. With the more bizarre of these varieties, it becomes apparent that most of these men are using the rings as a strange method of masturbation and not to enhance erections.

When the penis is caught inside such hard places, there is no easy solution. A team must be assembled to fix the problem. The fire department is usually called in to provide diamond drill bits and extraction materials. When such tools are used, tremendous heat is created by sawing these metals, so someone has to pour ice water on the heated body part while someone else runs the drill or saw. Others hold the penis or shields to protect the patient. After several hours of such metalwork, the steel eventually comes off. The patients hopes nothing else does. Everyone goes home with a great story, except the one member of the team who goes home with a sheepish grin and a black and blue penis.

Therefore, if you need a constriction ring, put out the twenty bucks or so for one of the commercial options listed above and keep off the list of infamous emergency room visits.

ALTERNATIVELY SPEAKING:
PRIMUM NON NOCERE

Natural foods and supplements were a way of life at Richard's house. His wife, Summer, made sure that they ate only organically grown foods. Everyone took *antioxidants* (derived from seaweed) and natural vitamins by the handful. The children were so accustomed to the practice that they didn't realize that some of their friends didn't do the same. With such a healthy lifestyle, it came as a shock to Richard and Summer when he began noticing less rigidity during erections.

The only explanation either of them could gather after looking into possible causes was that he must have been suffering from **performance anxiety**. Someone as young and healthy as Richard couldn't possibly have any physical reason to have erectile dysfunction, they reasoned. The only problem with this explanation was that Richard possessed as relaxed a personality as either of them could imagine. Not only was he relaxed at baseline, but also they were completely comfortable with each other sexually. Summer was well suited to avoid placing pressure on him, as she shared Richard's tranquil personality.

When things continued to worsen over the next few months, Summer researched options to improve erections naturally. She supplied her husband with ginseng, ginkgo biloba, and several different new vitamins. Oysters and organically grown eggs were added to their primarily vegetarian diet. Several spices that the health food store recommended were added to the diet as well. The change of pace to a diet that had gotten bland was fulfilling to the whole family, but not to Richard's erections.

He finally gave in and visited their family physician, Dr. White, to discuss the concerns. Everything seemed fine on examination, but a screening blood test panel showed that Richard's cholesterol and *triglycerides* (fats in the bloodstream) were sky high. The diagnosis became obvious—Richard's penis was the first organ to let him know it was not getting adequate blood flow due to hardening of the arteries (**arteriosclerosis**).

As it turns out, Richard had done everything right regarding diet and exercise, but had chosen the wrong parents regarding genes for high cholesterol and triglycerides. Richard's father had died of a massive heart attack in his early fifties, barely five years older than Richard now stood. Richard always (wrongly) assumed that his father died solely as a result of obesity and smoking—lifestyles that Richard had purposefully avoided.

The first recommendations Dr. White gave were to exercise and switch to a diet high in fruits and vegetables and low in fat and cholesterol. Unfortunately, Richard had already maximized those efforts even before receiving the doctor's advice in order to avoid his father's fate. Medications to lower the cholesterol and triglycerides were therefore in order.

When Richard returned home, Summer was incredulous. There was no way she was going to have her husband taking prescription medications. With a little research, she found that many physicians prescribed niacin, also known as vitamin B_3, for men like Richard. It was less than 10 percent of the cost of the prescription medications Dr. White had prescribed, and as a natural vitamin, it was in keeping with their philosophical viewpoint. The oysters were dropped, and niacin tablets were begun.

A repeat cholesterol level was indeed lower on the follow-up visit. Dr. White proudly noted that his prescription had worked well. Richard didn't feel the need to burst his bubble as long as the cholesterol was better, so he kept silent on the fact that he was taking niacin instead of the prescription Dr. White had written. However, Richard did have a new concern—diarrhea. Ever since the niacin had been started, bowel movements were loose and sometimes painful. With a diet that included maximum fiber intake, there was no reason for things to be anything but smooth. Dr. White was perplexed, and suggested consideration of yet another prescription medication, since the one he thought Richard was taking seemed to be causing some distressing side effects.

Americans spend more on complementary medical therapy ($13.7 billion) than they pay out of pocket for all hospitalizations ($12.8 billion). That indicates there is a huge amount of interest in alternative medicine. Contrary to popular opinion, the largest users are not the poor and uneducated. Quite the opposite, those spending cash on alternative medical treatments are more educated and have higher incomes than those who don't.[1]

Does that mean alternative therapy is more intelligent? Of course not. It just means that many people have a desire for alternatives to the mainstream treatments for all conditions, including erectile dysfunction.

Richard and Summer were therefore in good company in their quest to deal with health issues without using prescription medications. Their goal was entirely reasonable, as was the choice they made regarding niacin to lower cholesterol. Common medical practice indicated this was likely to work. The mistakes they made were twofold. First, they weren't open with Dr. White about the choice. That left him to make recommendations regarding Richard's health blinded to what was really going on. He could have made a major mistake in subsequently prescribing something that would have interacted with the alternative treatments he wasn't informed about. In some circumstances, serious or lethal consequences could occur.

The second mistake Richard and Summer made was in their assumption that something natural will be safer than something prescribed by a physician. As it turns out, Richard had side effects due to the natural treatment but not with the prescription he eventually decided to take. The opposite might have been true in another patient, but Dr. White's prescription was the right choice for Richard. His cholesterol is down and he continues to enjoy a healthy and active lifestyle. The erections aren't stellar, but they are adequate for the time being to satisfy both Richard and Summer.

One of the basic tenets of medicine is the Latin phrase, *primum non nocere*, meaning, "First, do no harm." Stated in a more modern phrasing, "The treatment should not be worse than the disease." The assumption of many people is that something natural can't be harmful, whereas something medical has to be. Remember that tobacco is a completely natural product—grown from the soil of Mother Earth herself.

ALTERNATIVE OR COMPLEMENTARY?

Differentiating between alternative and complementary medicine involves more than semantics. The word *alternative* means that something is used *in place of* established medical care. In contrast, the word *complementary* means that something is used *in addition to* mainstream therapy. The difference is huge. Alternative therapy is more likely to be dangerous, especially if used instead of proven medical treatments to manage life-threatening conditions such as cancer or cardiovascular disease. If proven treatments are foregone for unproven alternative therapy, disastrous consequences are risked. In contrast, complementary treatment is used to assist proven medical therapies. However, if not adequately tested scientifically, it could be very risky.

A good example of the difference would be when a patient has a heart attack and is prescribed aspirin and prescription medications known to decrease the chance of another, possibly fatal, heart attack. If he chooses alternative therapy, he would refuse the proven treatment and take something unknown, like tree bark or coffee enemas. Without the prescription medications, he will have a false sense of security right up until the next (and perhaps final) heart attack. In contrast, if he chooses complementary therapy, he will take the medical treatments known to lessen the chance of death. In addition, he might make dietary changes that improve overall health. He might add vitamins and antioxidants that *might* help augment the medications. In the worst-case scenario, they at least did no harm unless he took them in megadoses. *Primum non nocere.*

Therefore, complementary therapy may be safer than a truly alternative approach. A good example of a complementary treatment that is recommended by many urologists is the use of vitamin E and selenium for the prevention of **prostate** cancer. Based on observations that indicate these natural products may have a protective effect against the disease, I join many urologists in recommending that all men over the age of forty use these supplements (400 units of vitamin E and 200 micrograms of selenium daily). These natural complementary treatments are currently being investigated in formal fashion in the SELECT trial (see chapter 3, "A tomato a day keeps the urologist away").

Unfortunately, even complementary therapy has its risks as well, as some nonprescription items can affect how medications work. A good example is found in the intake of unusually large amounts of grapefruit (or its juice). Grapefruit contains a chemical that can block the liver enzyme P450, which is involved in drug metabolism. This can lead to toxic levels of many different types of medications by blocking the liver's ability to metabolize them.

Unfortunately, almost three-fourths of all patients who use complementary treatments do the same thing Richard did and fail to tell their physicians about alternative or complementary treatments they are using. This means that the physician is treating the patient without full information—no different than if the patient were on an undisclosed prescription drug that would interact with treatments. Therefore, complementary treatments should be taken into account by both the physician and patient in order to prevent disasters and achieve success.

NO REGULATIONS MEANS NO CLUE

Unconventional treatments often seem to make people feel more comfortable, even when their accompanying theories are silly.
—Edward W. Campion, "Why Unconventional Medicine?" 1993

The most worrisome problem with alternative and complementary therapy is the complete lack of reliable information available. Since most alternative medicine treatments are classified as food supplements instead of medications, they can make any claims they want and no one can legally refute them. Just like banana farmers could claim that eating the phallic-shaped fruit would lead to penile enlargement, the makers of *silver nitrate* or some tree bark product can claim it cures **impotence** (or cancer), and no one is able to confirm or deny the truth.

The reason these products aren't regulated or investigated is obvious. The companies can market and sell them with any claims they want as long as they keep them in the "supplements" category. Compared to the millions of dollars required for research necessary to bring a prescription drug to market, these agents can be on the shelves with the minimal cost of bottling, labeling, and shipping. More obviously, if these agents were to be studied scientifically, their claims would be subject to the same rigorous standards prescription medications must meet. Since it appears likely that many of them work by the **placebo effect** (if they work at all), there is no way most would pass the standard.

The placebo effect is a powerful tool. A placebo is something that is given to a patient that has no known effect on the condition being treated (often a sugar pill or other inactive ingredient). Interestingly, about one-fourth of people will experience improvement in a medical condition purely because they've been given something. In their mind, they *are* being treated, and the mind is a powerful broker. If convinced they should be getting better due to being given treatment, around one-fourth will say and believe they are, even if what they were given is a placebo. This effect can be especially pronounced for impotence treatments, because there is always at least some degree of psychological component involved.

The placebo effect is responsible for the fact that so many unproven treatments have testimonials to their effectiveness. Therefore, in proper medical studies, some patients are given the treatment, while a *control group* is given a placebo. Neither group gets to know if they are taking the drug or the placebo. If the symptoms of one-fourth of the patients in each group improve, a placebo effect is clearly the reason. However, if one-fourth of the patients in the placebo group are improved, but one-half of the patients receiving the tested substance are improved, the tested substance is clearly helpful for the symptoms in some patients with that condition.

A good example is found in the studies on Viagra. The trials used to obtain FDA approval for Viagra found that 25 percent of patients taking the placebo reported improvement in erections, whereas about 80 percent of those taking Viagra reported improvement. Therefore, the FDA agreed that the studies showed a clear benefit to Viagra in treating erectile dysfunction, so it was approved for use in the United States.

A LITTLE DOSE WILL DO YA?

Even if we did have evidence that alternative medications worked, the lack of regulation would still mean we have no idea how to use them. Manufacturers can label them as having an active ingredient without any quantification of the amount that is present. For example, the most popular alternative medicine treatment for prostate problems is *saw palmetto*, made from the bark of the small palm tree, *Serenoa repens*. This bushy plant was known for centuries as a "trash tree" that farmers tried to kill in order to keep it out of their fields. That all changed when it became popular as a prostate cure-all. With a mixture of traditional Native American medicine and the marketing machine of the complementary medicine industry, it has become perhaps the most widely used agent for prostate problems—prescription or not—in the world.

As it happens, the active agent in saw palmetto appears to have some effect that may actually help shrink the prostate.[2] The problem is that none of the versions on the market has a clearly defined amount of active agent. When tested scientifically, the amounts in various brands were all over the map. Some brands had several times as much concentration as others, although when you are buying pills on the Internet they all sound alike. Some brands barely had enough in them to justify noting it. Patients taking those brands were clearly receiving a placebo effect only, as they hardly got any of the active ingredient at all.[3]

If this only meant that we don't know whether an alternative treatment works or not, the only risk would be the waste of money for something that didn't work. Unfortunately, the risk is much greater, since these agents aren't inert at all. Many that seem as benign as grapefruit juice will interact with prescription medications to cause untoward effects. Many more have an effect on the cardiovascular system. Some may even increase the risk of death. *None of them is regulated.*

PC-SPES: COMPLEMENTARY MEDICINE TURNS SERIOUS

A recent example of the risk of alternative medicines was evidenced in the recall in 2002 of *PC-SPES*, a benign-sounding Chinese herbal product. PC-SPES is a "natural" product that appeared to cause regression of prostate cancer. So optimistic was the maker, BotanicLab, that it took the unusual step of having its product scientifically investigated by the University of California, San Francisco (UCSF).[4]

Researchers at UCSF were motivated to investigate PC-SPES based on the theory that its ingredients might have chemical activities similar to hormonal treatments already approved for prostate cancer (chapter 3, "A Nobel effort"). Early noncontrolled trials showed impressive results. As discussed above, the next step in figuring out whether these results were real or just due to the placebo effect was to begin a double-blinded, placebo-controlled trial.

Early in that trial, however, the California-based manufacturer voluntarily recalled the medication and closed shop. The product had been found to contain not only herbs but also the blood thinner *warfarin*: yes, the same warfarin that is used as a rat poison by farmers all over the world. Its blood-thinning capability is well known and has long been used as a prescription treatment for patients at risk of stroke or blood clots. However, it is such a dangerous drug that patients who use it must be monitored closely. These patients must have a blood test monthly to assure its level remains *therapeutic* (in the proper range). If the level goes too high, a fatal bleeding episode or stroke could occur. If too low, it might not prevent the problems it is prescribed for. Patients receiving warfarin in PC-SPES neither knew they were receiving it nor were monitored for appropriate dosing.

In addition, several lots of the product were found to contain *diethylstilbestrol (DES)*, the same hormone so reviled in the sixties because it caused *feminization* of male fetuses born to mothers who took it during pregnancy. This feminization made them develop female characteristics like small penises, undescended testicles (see chapter 3), or breast enlargement. Its effect on female offspring was even more alarming, as it caused a rare form of vaginal cancer when those babies reached adulthood—a long-term legacy.

DES itself is known to be an effective treatment for prostate cancer. Unfortunately, its side effects of stroke, blood clots, or other cardiovascular catastrophe have limited its usefulness (*primum non nocere*). Even so, it is sometimes worth the risk when the cancer is bad enough. The difference is that patients taking prescription DES are aware of that risk and make an informed decision under the guidance of their physician to accept it. In contrast, patients receiving DES in PC-SPES were taking a prescription cancer treatment with proven potentially fatal side effects without knowing enough to make such an informed decision. The irony is that warfarin is sometimes prescribed in order to prevent blood clots in patients taking DES. In a strange twist of fate, the two drugs contained in PC-SPES actually might have kept each other's side effects in check.

A sister product, *SPES*, was marketed by BotanicLab as an immune system enhancer. It sounded benign enough in the ads—until it was found to contain *alprazolam*. You might recognize that as the generic name of the prescription medication *Xanax*. It is one of the most effective tranquilizers on the market. In addition, samples were found to contain *indomethacin*, an anti-inflammatory drug used in humans and horses to treat arthritis.

The greatest danger of these drugs (warfarin, DES, alprazolam, indomethacin, and reportedly a couple of other possible medications) is that the recipients were taking something they believed to be safe and "natural," when in actuality they were taking prescription medications masquerading as nutritional supplements.

BotanicLab closed up shop and disappeared.

PROVEN COMPLEMENTARY OPTIONS

Just because something isn't an FDA-approved prescription medicine doesn't mean it isn't known to be beneficial. In Richard's case earlier in this chapter, niacin was a reasonable complementary medicine option to consider for lowering his blood pressure. This simple vitamin can be successful in many cases, even though it didn't end up being the right treatment for him.

As discussed earlier, we know that anything that promotes good overall health will improve the health of the penis. Therefore, a healthy diet combined with moderate exercise is clearly helpful for any man having erectile dysfunction (see chapter 10). For that matter, it's helpful for any man not yet having erectile dysfunction. Improving mental health is also undoubtedly helpful. This doesn't have to involve a therapist. It may mean getting some fresh air and sunshine. On the other hand, it might be as simple as dealing with chronic stresses that can paralyze you in more areas than those below the belt. Finally, getting enough rest to have energy left over for love is obviously worthwhile.

Studies have shown that a subset of men who take *L-arginine* may have improvement in erections.[5] Over one-third of men who took this *amino acid* (one of the building blocks that comprise all proteins) responded to this complementary treatment in a controlled medical study. Unlike claims made without evidence, there is actually a reason to believe this supplement might help some men with milder cases of erectile dysfunction. The reason L-arginine is thought to have an effect is that the men who respond have lower levels of **nitrates** and nitrites in their urine (indicating the body is getting rid of excess levels in normal men). Since L-arginine is involved in the **nitric oxide** chemical pathways that lead to a normal erection, restoring levels of this amino acid may be helpful for men who have a deficiency. That doesn't mean that all men should take it—just that a try is reasonable for some patients with minor difficulties with erections.

Sometimes, *not* doing something is the complementary treatment of greatest gain. Stopping cigarettes will make any treatment work better. Skipping that "one for the road" alcoholic drink that crosses the line from pleasantly relaxed to slurringly annoying might salvage the night.

Finally, anything that improves the quality of your relationship overall will improve your chance of success in bed. If your partner is working with you, she will be more likely to do whatever it takes to help stimulate you. More importantly, she will stick with you through whatever it takes to reach success.

All of these things are truly complementary to whatever intervention is required. Combining sensible nonmedical changes with medical assistance gives the best of both worlds.

VITAMINS: LIVING THE GOOD LIFE

> It is now known that all these diseases . . . can be prevented and cured by the addition of . . . the deficient substances, which are of the nature of organic bases, we will call vitamins.
>
> —Casimir Funk, 1912

The word *vitamin* comes from the Latin root *vita*, meaning "life." They are critical to life, but their exact role in your sex life is not clear. Note from the quotation above that they were only discovered less than a century ago. *Although there is very little scientific evidence to back up the claims*, several vitamins are touted for erectile dysfunction.

Vitamin B is actually a grouping of several different vitamins. Vitamin B_3 (yes, niacin) has been said to increase penile blood flow and orgasmic intensity. It's too bad Richard couldn't tolerate the side effects. Vitamin B_5 is said to improve **libido** and **orgasm**. Vitamin B_{12} has been touted for several sexual issues, especially to improve sperm function.

Vitamin C has been advocated as a cure for essentially every disease known to man due to its antioxidant capabilities, and erectile dysfunction hasn't escaped these claims. Its antioxidant qualities are said to prolong the life expectancy of everything in the body, including the penis. Another antioxidant, vitamin E, does seem to play a possible role in the management of **Peyronie's disease** (chapter 6) and may actually lessen the chance of developing certain cancers or cardiovascular diseases.

Zinc is a mineral found in substantial quantities in the reproductive system, especially the prostate. This finding has led many people to believe that zinc supplements can prevent prostate diseases and erectile dysfunction. Coincidentally, oysters are one of the highest natural sources of zinc, which gives some pseudoscientific credence to their status as aphrodisiacs. However, there is no scientific evidence that zinc matters regarding erectile dysfunction.

HERBAL REMEDIES

Herbs have been used for millennia to treat ailments before medicine existed. Herbal advocates reason that these treatments must work because they have been around for a long time. That logic makes no sense. People believed that the earth was flat for millennia, but that didn't make it so.

Black cumin seed comes from the *Nigella sativa* plant. It is the source of an oil famously found in the tomb of King Tutankhamen, used throughout the centuries as the *blessed seed* to improve erections and bring about childbirth. King Tut didn't feel so blessed, having died as a teenager without heirs. He hadn't even lived long enough to experience erectile dysfunction.

Bois bande is a tree whose bark is soaked in rum in order to be used as an aphrodisiac in the West Indies. Even if the bark was worse than its bite, the rum made for an interesting evening. *Broom rape* is a flower from the Far East believed to enable sexual conquest. *Damiana* is used in Central America as an aphrodisiac to inspire childbirth.

Ginkgo biloba is the ultimate wonder drug, if its advocates are to be believed. Its seeds and leaves are administered for almost any ailment. This makes it easy—no doses to remember—just give some to everyone and everything will get better. Although it appears to increase penile blood flow, it is also possible to overdose on ginkgo. Thereafter, the nausea, diarrhea, shock, and possibly death might make that newfound erection useless, so beware.

Ginseng is a highly sought-after root that is central to eastern medicine. An ancient Chinese emperor, Shen Nung, reported that it gave him warmth and sexual stirrings. His *Pharmacopoeia* is one of the oldest writings on medicines, advocating ginseng root to treat problems with just about everything, including the male root. An active ingredient, ginsenoside, appears to increase the release of nitric oxide (NO).

Kola nut is used in the Caribbean and South America as an aphrodisiac. *Mint* was recommended by Hippocrates as a "love brew." Rosemary, thyme, and saffron are all claimed to have a hormonal effect that improves libido.

Yohimbe is available in prescription form as the brand names *Yocon* or *Aphrodyne* (see chapter 12). However, it is also available in nonprescription capsules or as an extract of the bark of the African trees. However, just like its prescription form, it can have systemic side effects. These include central nervous system stimulation (anxiety) as well as panic attacks, hallucinations, elevated blood pressure, headache, or even death. The bark extract products are as variable in their concentration as saw palmetto is. Therefore a chemical that affects the blood pressure and cardiovascular system is ingested in these products in doses that can vary as much as twentyfold.

Arginmax is a product containing several of these agents, including L-arginine, ginkgo biloba, Korean ginseng, selenium, zinc, and vitamins A, C, E, and B-complex.

EATING FOR ERECTIONS

> Hence, a healthy and passionate man possessed of the necessary fecundating elements under the course of a proper Vaji Karana [aphrodisiac] remedy should cheerfully go unto and duly enjoy the pleasures of company with a woman.
>
> —Susruta, 1000 B.C.E., India

You are what you eat. That principle has led men to consume foods for centuries on the belief that certain cuisine increases virility. Casanova conquered a good portion of the female population of Europe with the help of as many as fifty *oysters* a day. With the popularity of zinc as a sex aid, a modern day (unproven) explanation for its reputation has re-emerged.

Artichokes were popular among the Romans for their arousing powers. *Sprouts* of innumerable vegetables have achieved legendary status for the power to heal all ills. As they are essentially emerging seeds, their symbolism may outpace their actual effects.

Asparagus, carrots, and *celery* share a shape that advocates feel raises their stock as aphrodisiacs. C. E. Hagdahl's book *Cooking as Science and Art* stated that celery is sexually exciting, but that the effect was diluted by boiling. Be careful, however. Quensel declared in 1809 that asparagus turns men on but turns women off. Some people have a genetic ability to smell asparagus as it passes through the urine as *asparagines,* but others can't smell this byproduct.

Garlic has proven effects on health, including controlling blood pressure and cholesterol. It was the basis of the love potions that spiced up the meals of such proven lovers as *Eros, Aphrodite,* and *Dionysus.* One ancient recommended crushing it into a love potion to rub onto the "unwilling" male member. It might be better on a bruschetta. Crowns of *fennel leaves* were worn by the Greeks during Dionysian festivals. It sent a signal akin to the modern-day practice of peeling the label from a beer bottle. Fresh fennel juice with milk is noted to be an aphrodisiac by the *Kama Sutra.*

Marc Antony did well by feeding grapes to Cleopatra, but the *Kama Sutra* recommends pomegranates as the sexual fruit of choice.

Spicing up your sex life might start in the spice shelf. *Clove* was advocated in 1642 by the Swedish herbalist Anders Rydaholm, who wrote, "If a man loses his virile power, he must cease drinking alcohol to replace it with milk spiced by means of five grams of cloves. That will strengthen it and will make him wish for his wife again." Wow, not only does it restore erections, but it also makes the patient's wife more alluring as well.

Nutmeg is said to do the opposite of asparagus. It arouses women, but leaves men dispassionate. That explains eggnog. *Pumpkin pie spice* is said to stimulate more than memories of Thanksgiving dinners past. This would likely be more effective on women than on men. *Cardamom* is a spice used in the Middle East for anything from coffee to dessert. It is thought to bestow power on anyone who consumes it. That power is thought to extend to one's manpower as well. Prepared in the sweet, sticky dessert *halwa,* it is the choice of the Indian movie hero to complete a romantic meal.

Ginger was rubbed onto any erogenous zone by the Roman intellectual Pliny the Elder. His *Natural History* was the first encyclopedia ever published. He got a little caught up in the aphrodisiac chapter (don't we all) and never achieved his goal of writing a tome that would "set forth in detail all the contents of the entire world."

Another holiday treat ingredient, *vanilla*, helps set the mood whether worn behind the ear or in a potion. Vanilla candles have a long history of setting the mood, although the effect of vanilla ingestion remains unproven. Moreover, the wholesomeness associated with vanilla may counter any perceived effect on *amour*.

HELP FROM THE ANIMAL KINGDOM

The powers ascribed to antlers and horns are notorious. Poaching for the purpose of obtaining them has led to the endangerment of several species. The Tibet red deer and all rhinoceros species are in danger of extinction due to the mass murder of these animals in order to harvest their horns.

Animal parts have been consumed in many parts of the world for their empowering effects. Ancient Egyptians ate crocodile penis, while ancient Eurasians preferred deer penis, which took much less effort. With no scientific evidence of which one is better—or even if either one works at all—stick with the deer if you are so inclined.

Spanish fly, mentioned earlier, is synonymous with aphrodisiac. Derived from the ground wings of the emerald-green *blister beetle* (*Cantharis vesicatoria*), it was touted as the salvation of elderly gentlemen as early as the first century, B.C.E. by such advocates as Hippocrates, Celsus, and Pliny the Elder. The Roman empress Livia slipped a little into the food of family members to drive them to indiscretions she could hold over their heads. Thereafter, she could blackmail them into doing her bidding in order to keep their secrets safe.

In 1772, the Marquis de Sade invented the sexual practice that bears his name when he spiced up dessert with Spanish fly. He added the beetle juice to aniseed sweets, knowing the prostitutes who came over for an orgy couldn't resist a little dessert after a romantic evening of flogging. However, putting a damper on the evening's festivities, most of the prostitutes began vomiting uncontrollably. In de Sade's day, flogging orgies weren't illegal, but poisoning was considered a grave offense, so he was forced to flee in the middle of the night. Having escaped capture, he was convicted in absentia and hanged in effigy—an orgy spoiled, if ever there was one.

HOMEGROWN HOMEOPATHY

> If you want to be sure not to reach threescore and twenty, get a little box of homeopathic pellets and a little book of homeopathic prescriptions.
> —Oliver Wendell Holmes, *Over the Teacups*, 1891

Homeopathy was founded by German physician and chemist Samuel Hahnemann about two centuries ago. It is based on the belief that trace amounts of a chemical can treat illnesses that they would otherwise actually cause if ingested in large doses. Tiny traces of substances are diluted many times over until the amount ingested would theoretically contain only a molecule or two of the agent. These minuscule amounts are believed by its followers to stimulate the person's immune system. The only problem is, there is no proof it works. However, as it continues to enjoy popularity in some crowds, the following is a list of touted homeopathic cures for sexual problems.

To treat poor erections, homeopathic followers would recommend *Agnus castus* (*monk pepper*), *Calcarea carbonica*, *Cannibas sativa*, *Caladium*, *Lycopodium clavatum*, and *sepia*. Performance anxiety is treated with *Argentums nitricum*, *Conium masculatum*, and *Kalium phosphoricum*. Psychogenic impotence is treated with just about any homeopathic remedy. **Rapid**, or **premature, ejaculation** is managed with *selenium* or *cinchona*, while excessive masturbation is controlled by *staphysagnia*.

The biggest problem with these homeopathic remedies is that they are all based on faith, without any investigation of their true physiologic actions. Interestingly, different homeopathy resources attribute different actions for many of these agents. That led Ambrose Bierce in 1906 to define a homeopathist as "the humorist of the medical profession." Therefore it is hard to draw any conclusions about potential effectiveness of homeopathic treatments.

KEY POINTS

- Vacuum constriction devices are noninvasive treatments options for erectile dysfunction.
- Constriction rings overcome venous leak syndrome and can augment erections for men needing just a little boost.
- Placing the penis through any nonexpandable device is likely to

make you the protagonist in a great story at the emergency room holiday party.
- Complementary treatments may play a role in dealing with erectile dysfunction, but care must be taken to understand how little is understood about them.
- Alternative remedies can pose a danger to your health.

12 When an Apple a Day Isn't Enough

Medical Therapy

For the millions of men who want to make love and can't, we are about to make your night.

—Hugh Downs, announcing FDA approval of Viagra

*M*y son, Jared, was ten years old when he gave us a shock one morning. His sister noted that it seemed his allergy symptoms were better than they had been the night before. "Your eyes aren't watering as much and you don't sound as stuffy," Katie observed. "You must have had a good night."

"Yeah, I had a *great* night," he assured in his sleepy, prepubescent voice. "I took a Viagra before I went to bed. It made my night *much* better."

My wife, Kathy, was apoplectic. "WHAT?!" she screeched in her most indignant Irish voice. "You—took—WHAT?" Maureen O'Hara couldn't have done it better. As the only urologist in the house, it was clear whose fault this was, as her gaze at me confirmed. "Did you hear what *your* son said?"

Redemption was gained with a combination of quick thinking and knowledge of pharmacology. "He took *Allegra*," I answered. "Not Viagra—*Allegra*. You know, the pill his pediatrician prescribed for allergies." Another crisis averted.

It's hard to believe that oral therapy for erectile dysfunction has been available for less than a decade. The other approved treatments in this book predated it. The Holy Grail for **impotence** treatment was to find a pill. That goal was met with rousing success in 1998 when Pfizer released Viagra. It was the most successful drug release in history, with sales of over a billion dollars in its first year on the market. Although sales cooled after the initial rush was satisfied, billions more have been sold since that time.

However, Pfizer's greatest achievement may not have been Viagra itself. The real world-changing event was bringing erectile dysfunction into the public eye. Prior to that time, men were much more hesitant to mention sexual difficulties to a physician. They were usually under the impression that surgery was the only thing that could be done. Until they were ready for an operation, they kept quiet.

That all changed in the explosion of a media frenzy. You couldn't turn on the television without hearing about erectile dysfunction. Suddenly, people were talking about erections at work, so it became acceptable to talk about them with a physician. As noted above, my ten-year-old son had heard about it.

This ushered the field of erectile dysfunction into a whole new era. Within twenty years, doctors had gone from telling men that the problem was in their heads to treating them right on the spot. No testing. No surgery. Just a prescription that fixed the problem by midnight.

SERENDIPITY SAVES THE DAY

> At the time, nobody yelled, "Yippee, never mind the angina, what about those erections!"
> —Ian Osterloh, M.D., Pfizer Laboratories

The story of Viagra's discovery is legendary. Scientists in 1986 at the Pfizer Corporation began looking into the enzyme *phosphodiesterase type 5* (*PDE-5*). Enzymes are chemicals that make physiological processes occur. They found that this one was involved in **vasoconstriction**, so they began working on a drug to block this action, which thereby could theoretically be used to treat cardiovascular diseases. After testing multiple agents, they identified **sildenafil** as the best one to block the enzyme.

Following some basic science animal studies and tests on healthy humans to assure its safety, they began randomized controlled trials in England (as discussed in chapter 12) to test their theory that the new drug could treat *angina*, the chest pain caused by severe heart disease. Because sildenafil could theoretically block arterial contraction and lower blood pressure to dangerous levels, they hospitalized the first test patients. Early results didn't show significant benefit regarding angina, but several of the volunteers reported an increased tendency to get erections. This was the only notable side effect identified in the early studies.

As you can tell from Dr. Osterloh's comments at the beginning of this section, this wasn't necessarily regarded as good news. The investigators were trying to save lives, so "the erections were a bit of a side issue," he remembers. It was only when the researchers realized that the new drug wasn't going to be the cure for heart disease that someone decided to look further into the erection issue.

Two of Pfizer's scientists had suspected this could be a side effect as early as 1991. Drs. Peter Ellis and Nick Terrett noted that sildenafil caused buildup of **cyclic GMP**, an enzyme that appeared to be related to the development of an erection. They theorized that this might make erections more likely, but saving lives seemed much more important. However, when it became clear this agent wasn't going to wipe out heart disease, these two researchers and some of the more open-minded leaders at Pfizer decided to pursue this intriguing side effect.

Randomized controlled trials began by giving the medication three times a day to men who were asked to watch erotic videos while hooked up to a **RigiScan** (as described in chapter 7). The **placebo effect** was clearly not responsible for the findings, as the men receiving the drug had an impressive response. Further studies showed that continual dosing three times a day was unnecessary. The medication could be taken as a single dose immediately before its effect was needed and it provided the same results.

PHOSPHODIESTERASE INHIBITION: STOPPING THE STOPPER

Recall from chapter 4 that **nitric oxide** is the *neurotransmitter* that releases cyclic GMP, which is the active chemical that causes penile blood vessels to open. This allows blood to flow into the penis to keep it full and under pressure. PDE-5 breaks down cyclic GMP, making the vessels close back down and allowing the penis to return to the flaccid state.

If things on the stimulating side of this equation are lacking, PDE-5 wins the battle and makes the erection go down. Viagra and the other drugs in its class are called **phosphodiesterase (PDE) inhibitors**. By blocking phosphodiesterases, PDE-5 inhibitors allow cyclic GMP to build up and keep the erection cascade in full bloom.

There are at least eleven phosphodiesterase enzymes in all, with each having a different effect in various organs. PDE-5 is the one most involved in erections. PDE-6 shares a similar chemical structure, so it also is inhibited by some of these agents. It is involved in retinal blood flow in the eye, so inhibition of PDE-6 explains a minor side effect (discussed later in this chapter.)

TAKING IT PROPERLY

"I need a penile implant," was the *chief complaint* listed on the information sheet Ron filled out during his initial consultation. That seemed to make evaluation and management of Ron's problem straightforward, but it seemed reasonable to further explore the situation. "I took a Viagra starter pack and it didn't help."

Upon further questioning, it became clear that his initial attempts were not well planned. The first two doses had produced no results. Of course, he took them before watching the baseball game. No effect. He attempted intercourse after taking the next two doses. Again, no effect. Finally, his primary care physician instructed him to take the final two tablets at the same time so he got the maximum dose—100 milligrams. Yet again, no effect. "I'm in that group that doesn't respond to medication," he lamented. "I need an implant."

Most men take their first doses of oral medications from sample packs. These became popular when the Pfizer Corporation made them available to essentially every American physician. Direct-to-consumer advertising made potential customers aware that all they had to do was ask their doctor and they would receive sample packs of six tablets. This worked well for many men, as the Viagra samples were 50 milligrams, a dose that was adequate for most men. If there was no response from taking the first two to four tablets, men like Ron were told to double the dose to 100 milligrams on the final attempt.

Due to increasing oversight by the Joint Commission on Accreditation of Healthcare Organizations (JCAHO) and other regulatory bodies, some physicians have abandoned providing samples. We have eliminated samples at the Cleveland Clinic Foundation due to the paperwork and regulations that must be observed. This has been frustrating to patients and physicians alike, but it became necessary due to the regulatory environment. Most private practice physicians still accept and distribute sample medications, however.

Almost half of men who fail to respond to medication may actually just be taking it incorrectly. Many of these men attempt intercourse too quickly, before the drug is in their circulation. If you pop the pill and immediately hop in bed, the medication is sitting in your stomach instead of in your penis. That won't work. Although the manufacturers of these drugs boast of quick onset, the surest way to get a good result is to take the medication at least an hour before you want it to be effective. Otherwise, the drug may take effect just as everyone becomes frustrated and falls asleep. A large meal slows this down even further (with or without alcohol).

Another mistake that some men make is in not realizing the way phosphodiesterase inhibitors work. They only allow accumulation of cyclic GMP as described above. Cyclic GMP only accumulates if it's being produced, and it's only produced in response to sexual stimulation.

Therefore, if you take oral medications and sit there waiting for something to happen, it could be a long night. This is actually an advantage of oral medications over injections or other treatments described in this book, as it mimics what happens during a natural erection. This is obviously an advantage for couples desiring a sexual experience that they regard as natural.

A final common reason men fail to respond to oral medications is due to taking an inadequate dose. There is a prejudice that lower doses are safer, so many physicians or patients aren't used to going up to maximal doses. If side effects of many medications occur, it happens almost as much at low doses. Therefore, you might as well reach an adequate dose. Many men who took medications from a sample pack but didn't respond will have success if educated by their physicians on taking the higher dosage while timing it early enough to have good blood levels by the time they attempt intercourse. Of course, this dosing must be under your physician's oversight and should never exceed the maximum dose. In addition, any dose of a PDE inhibitor can cause potential fatal interactions with **nitrates**, as discussed below.

A less common reason for men to not respond to oral medications is due to a temporary period following **prostate** surgery (as discussed in chapter 6) when the nerves are damaged but not destroyed. Oral medications may not cause an erection if used too soon following surgery, as the nerves are not fully recovered. Studies underway at the Cleveland Clinic

Urological Institute under the direction of Dr. Craig D. Zippe have found that it takes several months before oral medications work in most men. Therefore, if the initial attempts at taking them following prostate surgery aren't successful, you shouldn't give up. Rather, wait a few months and try again when the nerves have had more time to recover.

VARDENAFIL (LEVITRA)

Vardenafil is another PDE inhibitor similar to sildenafil (Viagra). The one potential difference is that it apparently has little effect on PDE-6, so doesn't have the minor visual side effects listed below. It was recently approved by the FDA for use in the United States to be marketed as **Levitra** (undeniably based on the root word *levitate*). There are indications that its onset may be quicker, which will be a selling point as well.

Although both manufacturers will make a big deal of the fine print, they appear so similar that they will be competing for the same customers. On potential advantage of Levitra may be that a large meal may not slow its absorption as much, although clinical experience will let us know if this is true. However, competition is always good in the marketplace, so both manufacturers will have to keep on their toes.

TADALAFIL (CIALIS)

Tadalafil appears to inhibit PDE-11 in addition to the PDE-5 and PDE-6 that sildenafil does. Its onset is slower than sildenafil and vardenafil, but it lasts two to three days. This means that it will be positioned as the "weekend drug." A dose Friday evening will cover both weekend nights and have enough leftover for a Sunday morning surprise. Couples who know their sexual activity is likely to be planned for these peak times will find it an easy way to have a boost to help them finish the marathon.

The disadvantage of tadalafil will be the same as its advantage—it may last too long. For men who are unlikely to go back for a repeat performance the following night (or day), this will be overkill. However, for the man taking his wife to New York for the weekend, it could be just the right thing.

SIDE EFFECTS

Phosphodiesterase inhibitors are among the safest prescription medications available. However, there is no medication that doesn't have side effects. Most side effects of these medications are related to their trait of dilating blood vessels. About 10 to 20 percent of men experience mild to moderate headaches due to the dilation of blood vessels in the head. Most men feel it's worth it. Flushing or redness occurs in about 10 percent, and nasal congestion occurs in 4 percent. Any drug can cause an upset stomach.

About 3 percent of men who take Viagra notice a blue tinge to their vision or enhanced light sensitivity due to the presence of PDE-6 in the retina. Sildenafil and tadalafil apparently also inhibit PDE-6. It is a strange, but minor, side effect that goes away as soon as the medication wears off. No permanent visual change has been reported. As noted above, vardenafil doesn't appear to affect PDE-6, so it doesn't cause this minor side effect.

Phosphodiesterase inhibitors also appear to lower blood pressure in men taking a group of medications called *alpha blockers* (including Hytrin, Cardura, and Flomax). This effect appears to be more significant for vardenafil, which therefore should not be taken by men who use alpha blockers.

A special warning about side effects goes to the man considering "sharing" medications. There have been some serious outcomes when men have shared their prescription with a friend. Face it, the friend may not want to admit that he takes nitroglycerin or similar nitrates for heart troubles. If you share with him, he could die. If he needs treatment, it should be under the care of a physician who can sort all this out, so don't fall into this potentially fatal trap.

WHAT ABOUT THE DEATHS?

Soon after the launch of Viagra, the news reports of patient deaths received intense media attention. There *were* deaths in men taking Viagra, but amazingly few for a medication known to affect the cardiovascular system. In fact, most deaths truly attributable to taking Viagra were in men who took it despite very clear warnings not to do so. These warnings concern the concomitant use of nitrates. Both these agents (PDE inhibitors and nitrates) dilate blood vessels independently. However, in combination they actually augment each other's effects on blood vessels. This leads to a dangerous dilation of blood vessels, thereby decreasing blood pressure to dangerous levels. In addition, these changes are not easily reversible, so the drop in blood pressure can (and has been) life threatening; in short, it can kill.

It is true that some men who take these medications die. However, this risk appears to be statistically about the same as the risk in men who don't use them. Sex involves significant physical exertion, so some men will have a heart attack during the exertion of intercourse with or without medications. This risk is said to be 142 in a million per year. That is less than the 200 in a million risk of dying in a motor vehicle accident during the year.[1] The risk of taking Viagra while driving has not been tested.

The only other drug interaction of note for these drugs involves the fact that they are metabolized by the liver using the cytochrome P450 enzyme. Therefore medications that compete for that enzyme can result in higher blood levels of the impotence drugs. These drugs include *erythromycin*, *cimetidine* (*Tagamet*), *ketoconazole*, and some *protease inhibitors* used to treat HIV.

The low risk of death appears to be the same with tadalafil (Cialis) and vardenafil (Levitra).

NITRATES

Most patients by now recognize the danger of taking Viagra and other phosphodiesterase inhibitors with nitroglycerin. However, nitrates come in different formulations. If you take *any* of these medications, you should *not* take Viagra or other phosphodiesterase inhibitors. Most of them are included in the following list:

> *Nitroglycerin* (brand names such as Nitrogard, Nitrostat, Nitrolingual, Nitrong, Nitroglyn, Nitro-dur, Nitrol)
> *Isosorbide* (brand names such as Imdur, Isordil, Sorbitrate, Dilatrate-SR)
> *Amyl nitrate* (inhalant, as discussed below)

Some patients try to take the position that they have nitroglycerin but don't ever use it, so it's okay to take these medications. This doesn't fly: a man either needs the nitroglycerin or he doesn't. If his cardiologist tells him that it's acceptable to discontinue it, fine. Otherwise, he shouldn't have a prescription for phosphodiesterase inhibitors, period.

POPPERS, PROTEASE INHIBITORS, AND PDE

"Poppers" are single-dose capsules or ampules of *amyl nitrate* or *butyl nitrate* that are mainly used in the nightclub scene to enhance sexual stimulation. These drugs are contained in glass or other breakable holders that can be broken (with a loud "pop," hence the name) in order to inhale their contents. Faithful users insist that poppers increase sexual stimulation and intensity of **orgasm**. They are favored mainly among the promiscuous, and appear to be used to overcome the natural **refractory period** between orgasms.

The active nitrates in these drugs share **vasodilation** properties with nitroglycerin, so using them in combination with PDE inhibitors can cause the same dangerous drop in blood pressure. When this occurs, users can die quickly in the nightclub bathroom. It was easy to predict that many people would combine a drug already being used to enhance sexual performance (poppers) with another drug that seemed to promise the same thing (Viagra). Unfortunately, because of this combination, there have been deaths reported in both the United States and Europe.

A popular but deadly cocktail used in this setting involves adding *crystal amphetamine* (no relation to amyl nitrate) to the other two. In combination, the poppers and PDE inhibitors cause **vasodilation**, whereas the crystal amphetamine tries to cause **vasoconstriction**. The vascular system doesn't know which way to go, but there is no way it is going to end up well. Therefore, when choosing which sex drug to take, you can choose a PDE inhibitor, which has been through the rigorous FDA approval process to assure maximum safety, or one of two illegal nightclub drugs known to cause death with misuse. The choice seems fairly straightforward.

Some AIDS patients are at risk of an especially dangerous mixture. *Protease inhibitors* prescribed to battle HIV interact with the PDE inhibitors because of their effect on the liver's *P450 3A4* enzyme. These medications will therefore cause enhancement of the PDE inhibitor effect. Poppers are especially popular within some segments of the gay community, where protease inhibitor use is also comparatively high due to increased numbers of AIDS cases. Therefore the risk of dangerous blood pressure drops is substantial when all these drugs are mixed. Other medications can affect the P450 3A4 enzyme, including *ketoconazole* and *erythromycin*. The result would be an alteration in different drug levels when this enzyme is altered.

WHICH DRUG IS BEST?

Although the makers of all three phosphodiesterase inhibitors feel theirs is best, the jury is still out on that question. Recall that all three enable erections due to similar chemical reactions and that the contraindications of all three are the same. The makers of Levitra believe their drug is faster in onset, so when the mood hits it can take effect without as much delay. However, this has not conclusively been proven to be true at this writing. The longer duration of action for Cialis may be better for men desiring intercourse on several occasions over a two- or three-day period. However, in the real world this may not be as important. In addition, the longer action means that any side effects may take longer to subside.

Our longest experience has been with Viagra, as millions of men have used the medication worldwide for several years. However, it appears that similar experience will accumulate with the other two medications, so differences may boil down to price and the preference of the patient and physician.

Finally, it is important to understand that similar-sized doses don't mean the same thing for different medications. Therefore, don't feel that a 50-milligram dose of one medication will necessarily be half as strong as 100 milligrams of another. They are different chemicals, so the numbers don't correlate when comparing drugs.

UPRIMA (APOMORPHINE)

Uprima is an **apomorphine** tablet dissolved under the tongue, which causes a rapid erection. It has been used in Eurasia and the Middle East for several years (also marketed under the brand name Ixense in some locations), but has had a difficult time receiving FDA approval for use in the United States. Apomorphine has been used for multiple applications since 1869 and is used in veterinary medicine to induce vomiting in animals that have swallowed toxic substances. It is not surprising, therefore, that over 10 percent of men using Uprima complained of nausea. This makes its use in the throes of passion a bit limited. Those experiencing this side effect have to hope that their penis comes up before their lunch does. Nevertheless, since it can be used in men unable to take PDE inhibitors due to nitrate requirements, many men around the globe benefit from this drug.

Uprima works in a very different manner than the PDE inhibitors. It affects the dopamine receptors in the brain that are involved in pleasure signals of the central nervous system. This makes it the only *centrally acting* (brain level) agent for erectile dysfunction.

VASOMAX (PHENTOLAMINE)

Phentolamine is used for penile injections (see chapter 13). Its release as a pill named *Vasomax* has been held up for further animal studies required by the FDA. It was developed by the Zonagen Corporation and licensed to large pharmaceutical company Shering-Plough. It is unclear what the status of Vasomax is at this point.

BARKING UP THE WRONG TREE

The bark of the central African *Paysinystalin yohimbe* tree has been used as an aphrodisiac for centuries. The active agent is believed to affect chemical receptors in the brain that contribute to sexual stimulation. Unfortunately, this has not been proven scientifically.

We know that it works in the brain and not the penis because of one of Dr. Giles Brindley's experiments. He injected **yohimbine** into the penis without response (Dr. Brindley is the star of chapter 13 for his work with penile injection therapy). We also know that it works in the brain due to its side effects, which include anxiety, nausea, palpitations, tremors, and elevated blood pressure (in the arteries, not the penis).

TREATING DEPRESSION AND ERECTILE DYSFUNCTION

Trazadone is an antidepressant that isn't too popular these days due to the introduction of the newer group of antidepressants called SSRIs. However, it has a history of causing **priapism** (painful, prolonged erection) in some men who took it, so it clearly has some effect on erection. Intriguingly, it has even been shown to cause priapism of the clitoris in women taking the drug. (The penis and **clitoris** are exactly the same in the developing fetus as discussed in chapter 8. The phallus grows more in a man, but it has all the same parts in the woman, only smaller).

More recent experience has found little benefit to trazadone regarding erections. Since we have better drugs available, its use for erectile dysfunction has been relegated mainly to historical interest.

TESTOSTERONE REPLACEMENT

Tim complained to Dr. Black that his **libido** was poor. In addition, he had no energy and was tired all the time. He thought it was due to overworking, but when he retired he found the symptoms just continued to worsen. That meant he couldn't blame his killer schedule any longer.

They agreed that signs of depression were present, and Tim was started on an antidepressant. Although his mood improved a little bit, there was no change in libido. Amanda, though understanding, pointed out that Tim no longer initiated intercourse. This was a big change from recent years, when Tim usually was the one asking for more. Fortunately, Tim was always willing and able when she made advances, although not with the same fervor as before.

After a month on the antidepressant, Tim told Dr. Black that he didn't think it was really solving his biggest complaint. Other than mild improvement in his demeanor, things seemed unchanged. A **testosterone** blood test was performed, showing that Tim's hormone level was exceedingly low. Further blood tests found that the cause was a small tumor in Tim's *pituitary gland* (as discussed in chapter 6). The tumor was not cancerous and was easily managed with surgery.

Unfortunately, Tim's testosterone level still didn't return to normal due to permanent damage to the pituitary gland. However, testosterone gel was prescribed and within a couple of weeks his libido was back to normal. Amanda didn't have to be the instigator very often thereafter.

As we have discussed, for most of medical history, impotence was believed to be mainly "in the head." The only medical treatment available for years was, therefore, testosterone replacement.

Testosterone replacement is like pouring water into a glass. If the water (or testosterone) is low, adding some will make a difference. However, there is no benefit to adding more once the water (or testosterone) level reaches the top. That means that the testosterone level in the bloodstream should be measured before empirically giving testosterone. If this level is normal, the risk of giving replacement outweighs the benefit.

Since testosterone is a normal hormone, bringing it up to normal levels shouldn't cause any problems. However, dosing beyond normal levels can cause it to stimulate the growth of prostate tissue (as discussed in chapter 3). That discovery allowed scientists to block the hormone in order to control prostate cancer. It also came to mean that testosterone in normal amounts isn't a problem, but if a person has prostate cancer or other prostatic diseases (such as enlargement), administering testosterone will cause the disease to progress more rapidly.

Some men confuse these facts and think that testosterone *causes* prostate cancer. On the contrary, we know that it is only a growth factor for the disease. A good analogy is that testosterone is like fertilizer in the garden. You can put as much fertilizer as you want onto the garden, but it won't make weeds appear. However, if weeds are present, fertilizer will make them grow faster. Likewise, testosterone won't make prostate cancer appear. However, if cancer arises on its own, testosterone will make it grow like a weed. For that reason, men receiving testosterone replacement must be screened carefully for prostate cancer (as discussed in chapter 3). If there is any suspicion of this disease, hormone replacement must be discontinued until the doctor is absolutely sure there is no prostate cancer.

In addition, doses above normal physiological levels can suppress the *pituitary gland*, which stimulates normal testicular function in the first place. This can lead to infertility (sterility) from blockage of sperm formation. As athletes who take excessive testosterone know, it can also cause the blood to thicken and the testicles to thin.

The traditional manner in which testosterone is administered is by injection every two to four weeks. This episodic dosing pattern means that a huge dose is present for the first few days but slowly decreases until the next shot is given. That creates a very uneven hormone level in the bloodstream, which can cause an uneven response. Slow-release patches and skin creams that allow sustained, stable blood levels have recently been perfected.

The only route of testosterone administration that we don't recommend is orally. Testosterone pills have to pass through the liver as they are absorbed from the intestines. This *first-pass effect* through the liver renders most of the drug metabolically inactive. The temptation to simply increase the amount administered orally should be avoided, as large doses are toxic to the liver and could lead to hepatitis, jaundice, and liver cancer.

Ketoconazole is a particularly effective blocker of testosterone that is often prescribed for fungal infections of the skin or nails. Since it is prescribed for such seemingly benign conditions, many patients forget to even list it when asked about medications. This is unfortunate, because stopping it can yield a rapid return to normal testosterone levels.

TOPICAL DRUGS

Medications that are rubbed onto the skin are called *topical*. The concept makes a lot of sense, as they are applied directly to the body part where they are needed. The concept doesn't always hold up, however, since medications applied in this manner also get absorbed into the blood vessels of that skin. This means they end up going into the systemic circulation. Despite this limitation, several companies are still trying to make the concept work. Most of the medications used are the same ones administered via other routes, as discussed below.

PROSTAGLANDIN E1

Prostaglandins are a large group of chemicals originally discovered in the prostate (thereby, the name) in the early twentieth century by Sune K. Bergstrom. He shared the 1982 Nobel Prize with Bengt I. Samuelsson and John R. Vane, who identified critical functions that prostaglandin performed all over the body, not just in the prostate.

One of these functions involves vasodilation, which is why they have been of interest to those working on treatments of erectile dysfunction. The best and safest vasodilator is **prostaglandin E1**. This version has been used successfully for several years when injected into the **corpora cavernosae** (as discussed in chapter 13). When applied to the skin, only limited amounts make it inside the corporae, so success hasn't been as good.

Studies continue for its possible future marketing as *Topiglan* (made by MacroChem, Lexington, Massachusetts) or in combination with *prazocin* as *Alibra* (made by Vivus, Mountain View, California). At this writing, both manufacturers are still attempting to receive FDA approval.

NITROGLYCERIN: NOT TONIGHT, DEAR, I HAVE A HEADACHE

Since nitroglycerin is widely known as a vasodilator, it makes sense that rubbing it on the penis would produce an erection. Well, the rubbing may help, but the nitroglycerin is absorbed more into the bloodstream than into the penis, so most of its effect is systemic. That means that a small improvement in erections will occur, but systemic side effects make it not worthwhile. All the vessels in the body dilate, which causes lowering of blood pressure. When nitroglycerine causes dilation of the vessels inside the head, it just puts pressure on the brain, leading to a rousing headache.

Since the nitroglycerin is on the penis, some of it will rub off in the **vagina**. The vagina is comprised of the type of tissue that readily absorbs medications. Therefore the partner gets a pretty good dose as well. Although things might start off well, the cause of coitus interruptus might honestly be, "Not tonight, dear, I have a headache."

OTHER TOPICAL AGENTS

Interest in developing a treatment that could easily be rubbed on remains high. Topical **papaverine**, another drug that is beneficial when injected into the penis, is undergoing trials. It causes some **tumescence** (erection) when placed on the skin, but not enough. *Minoxidil* in combination with a hot pepper (*capsaicin*) seems to have some dilating effect as well. At the time of writing, none of these agents have received FDA approval.

KEY POINTS

- The introduction of Viagra as the first effective oral agent to treat erectile dysfunction revolutionized the treatment of this problem. Its impact on sexual behavior has been compared to the introduction of oral contraceptives.
- Phosphodiesterase inhibitors such as Viagra, Levitra, and Cialis are effective and safe when used appropriately.
- Taking any phosphodiesterase inhibitor with nitrates, however, can be potentially fatal.
- Restoring testosterone levels to normal can be effective therapy if a man suffers from a deficiency.
- Several alternative medications are being investigated and considered for approval by the FDA.

13 Penile Injection Therapy

Rise and Shine

He that sweetest rose will find,
Must find love's prick and Rosalinde.
—Shakespeare, *As You Like It*, act 3, scene 2

*I*t's almost impossible to shock urologists, but Dr. G. S. Brindley succeeded when he introduced penile injection therapy to the American Urological Association (AUA) meeting in 1983.

"Immediately before I came to the podium," he said, "I injected my own penis with a new treatment for impotence. I'd like to show you my results."* The audience woke up when Dr. Brindley unzipped his pants, pulled the proof out, and walked down the center aisle. He invited participants to examine his upstanding evidence. After witnessing an obviously foolproof treatment for performance anxiety, the following speaker could only lament, "I have a hard act to follow."

Brindley's treatment, now called **intracorporeal pharmacotherapy (ICP)**, changed everything. If men were willing to inject themselves in the penile shaft with a medication, most were able to have fully functional erections within minutes.

---

*As usual, on long days at medical conferences, no one was paying that much attention before this, so we don't really know his exact words.

PENILE INJECTION THERAPY: THE PROCEDURE

The idea of placing a needle into the penis is not something most men relish. Fortunately, a very small "diabetic" needle is all that is required. More importantly, the needle is not placed in the sensitive part at all. The injection site is at the base of the penis where it exits the body—a location no more sensitive than the part of the arm where blood is usually drawn. So although penile injection usually hurts less than a blood test, the recipient is left much more satisfied. The technique is so easy that most men learn it in one or two teaching sessions. Thereafter, the patient can self-inject any time he wants to have an erection—ready for any occasion.

How does it work? Medications are injected into the **corporal bodies** (see chapter 2) as shown in Figure 6. This causes dilation (opening) of the

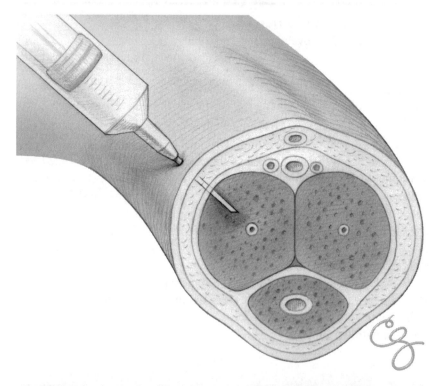

Fig. 6. Proper needle placement into the corpus cavernosum near the site where the penis exits the body wall.
(Illustration courtesy of the Vivus Corporation, Mountain View, California.)

arteries to the penis so the shaft fills under pressure within minutes. This filling is what makes the penis become firm and erect normally.

Remembering there are two corporal bodies (see illustration) you might wonder if two injections are required. No, these bodies openly communicate so the medication automatically causes filling of both.

Although Dr. Brindley introduced the procedure to the urological world, the concept of injecting the penis is actually older than urology. French pathologist Regneri de Graaf observed in 1668 that injecting blood or water (reports conflict on which one he used) into the penis of dead men caused postmortem erections. His findings were not clinically useful at the time—no one alive would allow him to inject blood into the penis, and none of his dead patients needed erections.

The availability of oral medications made this formerly first line therapy much less popular, since popping a pill sounds better to most men that injecting the penis. However, for men who can't or don't want to take oral medications for the reasons discussed in chapter 12, injection therapy is an excellent alternative.

CAPITALISM HITS BELOW THE BELT

In the twentieth century, a surgeon named Virag made a serendipitous finding when he accidentally injected medication into a penile artery during surgery. He and the operative team noticed a pup tent rising under the surgical drapes. Dr. Alvaro Latorre subsequently injected several different medications into his own penis unsuccessfully but foresaw value in the technique. He obtained U.S. patent number 4,127,118 in 1977 and sold it to a group of nonurologists known as Men's Health Resources. When the treatment was refined to success by the nineties, this organization sent letters to essentially every American urologist demanding royalty payment of $300 or more. They threatened patent litigation against any urologist prescribing penile injection therapy if payment was not made.

Since the AUA had supported ICP as an acceptable form of **impotence** treatment—realistically the only successful option available at the time—this created a storm of controversy. It is not known how many urologists actually paid the ransom, but apparently not many, since I can't find anyone who will admit doing so. Nevertheless, the idea that a medical procedure could be patented—and withheld from appropriate patients—challenged medical moral boundaries.

The whole issue disappeared when the Upjohn Company sought FDA approval for their brand of penile injection, **Caverject**. As part of their approval process, they reportedly made a deal with Men's Health Resources that put the patent controversy finally to an end.

Ending the patent controversy was the good news; money was the bad news. Prior to that time, there were two main medications available for penile injections, neither of which was approved for impotence.* The first option at that time was **papaverine**, used mainly as a cardiovascular medication. The maker of papaverine felt legally at risk by its medication being used off-label in this manner, so it took a public stance that its medication was contraindicated for penile injection therapy. Their product insert put it in black and white. This meant that if any patient had any problem with the treatment, the manufacturer was on record as saying the urologist was at fault. The lawyers loved this; the urologists knew it was the end of papaverine for the foreseeable future.

The other medication available then was **alprostadil**, an excellent medication for penile injection that was sold inexpensively in multiuse bottles. However, after the brand-name version of alprostadil (Caverject) received FDA approval, generic alprostadil was no longer available. Overnight, the cost for a single penile injection went from a few dollars to over twenty dollars. If used with any regularity, few patients could tolerate this cost. With papaverine and generic alprostadil suddenly both unavailable, penile injection therapy's role in impotence treatment started to go downhill quickly. Those who could afford Caverject did well, but many patients had to stop treatment because of cost. Fortunately, with time other manufacturers have filled in the gaps, so we now have several options from which to choose.

THE MEDICATIONS

Almost every **vasodilator**† known to man has been used, but currently there are mainly three medications being prescribed. The most common is still alprostadil. It is now available generically or in single-use packs under the brand names Caverject and **Edex**. The same chemical, they are both

---

*The FDA approves medications for very defined indications. Once approved, however, physicians are allowed to prescribe the medication for any purpose they feel appropriate. This so-called off-label prescribing is very common for most medications.

†Vasodilators are medications that cause blood vessels to expand. By increasing the open channel through a blood vessel, more blood flows through.

packaged with the medication, syringe, alcohol pad (to sterilize the skin), and instructions. Although both manufacturers say theirs is better or more convenient, they are virtually identical medications with slightly different syringe systems. Both are self-contained and require mixing the medication immediately prior to injection. Each maker has developed unique injection systems to simplify use.

The second medication is our old standby papaverine. Papaverine is once again readily available in multiuse bottles. It is often mixed with the third drug, **phentolamine**, in order to minimize side effects and cost. Phentolamine by itself is not very effective, but it helps the other two to work better and in lower doses.

Patients currently can take either the brand-name options (Caverject or Edex) or the generic versions of one, two, or all three medications. When combinations ("**bi-mix**" or "**tri-mix**") are used, the pharmacy usually prepares specific combinations prescribed by the urologist.

NEWER DRUGS

More recently, a new drug named **forskolin** has been used in some patients who don't tolerate the traditional medications. It is a natural product derived from the root of the Asian plant *Coleus forskolii*. This has reportedly caused less pain than the standard medications and can be used in a "quad-mix" with the other drugs. The *natural* source of this one might make it attractive to those desiring only natural treatments, although nature may not have envisioned this plant being injected into the penis.

Moxisylyte is very safe, rarely causing side effects, but it is less potent than the other available agents. *Vasointestinal peptide* is effective, but mainly in combination with phentolamine. Vasointestinal peptide has been humorously abbreviated VIP, which clearly doesn't mean "very impotent person." Several other drugs, including *CGRP, linidomineis*, and *sodium nitroprusside* can work, but none of them has matched the three primary drugs described above.

SUCCESS WITH INJECTION THERAPY

After surgery to remove a large cancerous tumor of his colon, Anthony was relieved to get the report that he appeared to be cured. Unfortunately,

removal of the tumor also necessitated removal of the pelvic nerves responsible for erections. Oral medications were unable to overcome such extensive nerve damage. His colorectal surgeon arranged a consultation to consider alternatives. When hearing that ICP was probably the best option for
him, Anthony's grimace was unambiguous. He left the first visit discour-
aged about his sex life. A longtime needle-phobic, the idea of a needle—no
matter how small—wasn't something he could face. Also unwilling to consider surgery to place a penile prosthesis, he chose to forego treatment.

Several months later he returned, probably to find out if any new discoveries had arisen since the initial visit. Disappointed that there weren't,
he gave in and considered ICP. Knowing he was so anxious about the
needle, I went ahead and injected him in the office that day just so he
wouldn't have time to back out. Before he had a chance to get more
nervous a sample vial of Caverject was prepared and aspirated into the
small syringe. Seconds after he lowered his pants, I had swabbed the base
of his penis with alcohol, placed it on stretch, and pricked the appropriate
site. A quick push on the plunger injected one milliliter of Caverject pain-
lessly. Just as quickly as it started, I gave him a cotton swab to put pressure
on for a few seconds and walked out to see my next patient. "Feel free to
make yourself comfortable," I told him on the way out to give good test
results to the man nervously pacing the floor awaiting **biopsy** results in the
room next door.

The ten minutes it took to calm down the next patient were all it took
to perk up Anthony. "How is it working?" I asked coming in the door. He
was speechless. In the sterile, daunting atmosphere of the Urological Institute, he had an erection that matched anything from his youth. With his
wife at home, a thirty-minute drive away, while he stood in the office
sporting the first erection he'd had in months, he looked a little confused.
"Do you think that'll work?" I asked.

"I'll let you know tomorrow. I'm outta here," he replied on the way
toward the waiting room.

Injection therapy usually works in motivated patients who are willing to
tolerate the needle. The treatment in India has been nicknamed *PIPE*, an
acronym for *Pharmacological Inductor of Penile Erection*, which does justice in its description of the results. Most patients attain erections capable
of penetration if the dose is adjusted to an adequate level. "Sticking" with
it is another matter.

Almost half of all men who start using ICP will stop within a year for various reasons. Some dislike the lack of spontaneity. Some just don't like needles. Some decide other options better suit their needs.

A number of men reach a point they no longer require therapy at all, often because they no longer wish to be sexually active. Men may get older or otherwise infirm and no longer desire sex, impossible as it may sound. Others lose their partners through death, illness, or divorce. A great number of men simply want to know that they could achieve erection again. Once reassured of their abilities, a significant number of them simply find that they and their partners really didn't want intercourse; they simply needed to know it was an option.

JUST WANTING TO KNOW I'M STILL A MAN

Harold is a seventy-eight-year-old retired farmer with prostate problems. I routinely ask men whether they have difficulties with erection, and as is common, Harold said he hadn't really been able to have a full erection in years. Oral medications were contraindicated (as discussed in chapter 12) because he took nitroglycerin occasionally for angina, so I started him on ICP.

At his next visit, Harold and his wife were both almost giggly about their renewed sex life. He requested refills and left very happy. However, a few months later he admitted they had used the injections infrequently. After an initial period, they realized their marriage was fine without intercourse, and neither of them really enjoyed it as much as they had previously.

I was intrigued when he wanted another refill. "Why?" I had to ask.

"I just want to know that *if* I want to, I can," he replied. "I just want to know that I'm still a man."

I saw no reason to talk him out of it.

NOW TELL ME THE BAD PART: SIDE EFFECTS

Like any medical advance, penile injections have some side effects patients must consider when beginning therapy. The most significant one is **priapism** discussed earlier. This is a prolonged erection that doesn't go down within a period of time, usually defined as four hours. The word comes from the god *Priapus*—the fertility god—always portrayed with a permanent erection protruding out of his toga. For men who have not been able to get an erection at all, an unending erection seems preposterous. This is fortunately very rare, but if not reversed within a few hours the penis actually becomes damaged and develops scarring, or **fibrosis**. Thereafter, the anatomy of the penis may be so damaged that erections are impossible.

Occasional patients with priapism will respond to oral medications like pseudoephedrine or other similar agents (*vasoconstrictors*, the opposite of vasodilators). Most, however, must urgently see the urologist. The priapism can then usually be reversed by injecting a vasoconstrictor into the penis. Rarely the condition won't reverse at all and surgery may be required to open the penis and release the pressure.

For obvious reasons, then, we start with low doses. If the initial dose isn't successful, don't despair. We can usually **titrate** upward to the right dose, which means slowly increase the dose until the desired result if found. We rarely see priapism if done in this manner. Not surprisingly, most cases of priapism are just due to an excessive dose. In the past decade I have seen only two cases of priapism following ICP. Both were in men that intentionally exceeded their prescribed doses. Be careful what you ask for.

Men who are at increased risk of priapism include those with sickle cell disease, hemophilia, and leukemia. Anyone with these conditions or those with a history of priapism should avoid injection therapy.

The biggest advantage of alprostadil over papaverine is the much lower risk of priapism. That's the good news. However, infrequent patients develop severe pain from the alprostadil itself (not the needle) that persists until the medication wears off. Fortunately, alprostadil wears off in one to two hours, and the pain resolves completely. Although decreasing the dose by using the tri-mix might allow some of these men to tolerate alprostadil, most will have to switch to papaverine. Adding a local anesthetic into the injection can also help sometimes.

Almost all other ICP complications come from the needle itself. Sticking a needle anywhere can cause bleeding, bruising, infection, scarring, or pain. The penis is no different; we're just more protective of it.

Scarring from repeated injections on one side of the penis may make that area less elastic. That section will then stretch less than the opposite side during erection, leading to curvature (similar to the situation found in **Peyronie's disease**). Alternating sides each time you inject will keep any scarring symmetrical, assuring a straight shooter. Very rare cases of corporeal fibrosis have been reported, where the penile tissue develops widespread scarring. Papaverine is more likely to cause fibrosis. This rarely occurs, but it is a good reason for the urologist to examine you on a regular basis to check for any early signs of a "permanent woody." Unfortunately, this is more like cork than wood and yields very unsatisfactory results. If this is beginning, most patients should change to another form of therapy.

Very rare cases of liver damage from papaverine entering the bloodstream have caused some concern. This has not been noted with alprostadil. Obviously, sharing needles should absolutely not be done. First, it risks infections, including AIDS and hepatitis. Second, a needle that's been in your penis is somewhat personal.

Limiting injections to one per twenty-four-hour period minimizes the chance of any of these complications occurring. Face it—no one really needs it more often than that.

PRIAPISM: TOO MUCH OF A GOOD THING

Ted is a fifty-two-year-old divorced respiratory therapist. He has always described himself as "sexually active," often with serial one-night stands. As he has "matured," his ability to perform nightly has waned, and Viagra caused him intolerable headaches.

He started using ICP injections when an older friend lent him a dose. Impressed by the results, he convinced me to prescribe them for him by exaggerating his difficulties obtaining erections. Because of his young age, I started him on low-dose alprostadil and gave him the usual instruction never to take more than one dose in any 24-hour period. As I also instruct any patient, I told him to report any erection lasting more than three to four hours.

The next time I heard from Ted was the Monday morning after his fifty-third birthday, when he called requesting pain pills for an erection he said had persisted since Friday afternoon. He had injected after work and twice more before sunrise. He found it fun at first, proving to his "dates" that a fifty-three-year-old man could perform essentially around the clock.

By Sunday the "dates" got bored and left. The erection didn't. Too embarrassed to admit what he'd done, Ted tried ice packs, showers, and masturbation—every method he knew to get rid of an erection.

When he called Monday morning, I instructed him to come in immediately. He refused because he had to work. By Tuesday, the erection was almost gone. I made it clear that because of his misuse of the medication I would not prescribe it for him again.

Another urologist that didn't know Ted's history of misuse prescribed the same treatment a week later, but Ted discovered that the priapism had caused irreversible damage to the erectile tissue of the penis. Unable to have an erection any other way, he asked each of us to place a penile prosthesis to overcome the damage he had done to himself through his poor decision-making. Both of us wisely said no.

WHICH MEDICATION IS RIGHT FOR YOU?

Deciding which medication to use can be tricky. As cost is often an issue, buying it in bulk and drawing up individual doses into a syringe is clearly the least expensive option. If you are one of the fortunate men whose insurance covers ICP, you may actually be better off using the brand names. Because only Caverject and Edex are FDA-approved for impotence, many insurers will cover these but refuse to cover the generics, including bi-mix and tri-mix. Economic logic is missing but that's typical of big insurance companies. Many insurers have a *formulary*, or a list of medications they will pay for, that may only cover one of these two medications. Since Caverject and Edex are virtually the same chemical, use whichever one your insurance will cover.

When the cost comes out of pocket, the mixes are the way to go. With the savings, you can buy a bottle of wine and a Barry White CD to help make the evening everything you've built up to.

Since the mixes are not FDA-approved for impotence, some patients are uncomfortable using them "off-label." This clearly must weigh into your decision on whether to take them in this form. Remember, though, that they are FDA-approved for general vasodilation and have been used now for twenty years with great success (recall Dr. Brindley's victory march). If you and your urologist can get over this issue—and most urologists have—huge savings are in store.

You probably wonder why generic alprostadil, papaverine, and phentolamine aren't FDA-approved for impotence. The answer is money. The FDA approval process would cost the companies millions of dollars. Once approved, they wouldn't get any more prescriptions for this use than they are getting now. It's simple math.

WHEN IS GENERIC MORE EXPENSIVE?
WHEN INSURANCE IS INVOLVED

Tom began using ICP after prostate cancer surgery in 1994. When Caverject was released, he was so upset at the increased cost over his generic alprostadil that he stopped therapy for a short period. He resumed use of the generic as soon as it again became available.

When he turned sixty-five, he signed up for a Medicare supplemental insurance policy with prescription drug coverage. While trying to fill a generic alprostadil prescription, he found that it was not covered. Therefore, although the actual cost of Caverject was several times higher than generic alprostadil, I switched Tom to Caverject because his monthly co-pay was only $15 for up to ten single-dose packs.

The economics were straightforward to Tom. The insurance company could save a lot of money by paying for the generic alprostadil, but because of their formulary rules Tom saved money while the insurer paid more.

TECHNICAL TRICKS

The technique is readily learned with no previous medical training. Caverject and Edex supply a handout in the single-use packaging that walks you through. We always go through the steps in the office with patients, and preferably their partner, the first time. Most can do it on their own after that.

Those choosing the generic options need a little more hands-on teaching. The urologist may do this, but many large group practices have trained **impotence coordinators** or nurses that spend most if not all of their workdays doing impotence teaching. These individuals can be extremely useful in all phases of treatment. They can also help patients assess other options that might better meet their needs.

Since this procedure should be learned from a professional, I won't give step-by-step instructions. However, if you're already using penile injections, there are some tricks that can help:

1. *Pull firmly* on the penis. Remember junior high school? It won't pull off. If not stretched, it will flop around as the needle is inserted, and accuracy will suffer.
2. *Put it in.* Many men hesitate as they place the needle. Just like pulling off a Band-Aid hurts much more if you hesitate, ICP hurts more if you just sit there tapping the penis with a needle.
3. *Push it in.* Once the needle is in, inject the medication quickly as well. The longer time the needle is inside the penile shaft, the more time for it to dislodge.
4. *Relax.* As long as you have the correct dose, there's not much that

you can do seriously wrong. If the needle goes in the wrong place, nothing will happen. If you don't get within the corporal bodies the medication will go into your bloodstream and no erection will occur. At worst, you might get a little bit flushed, but your whole body won't get stiff. If you get too far on the underside of the penis, the medication will go into the **urethra**. You might urinate it out, but that's okay. You'll live to fight another day—or night.

5. Most importantly, *start slowly*. We can always add more, so if the first attempts aren't successful, just follow your urologist's advice and work up to your proper dose. Once injected we can't take it out, so don't swing for the fences your first time up to bat.

6. *Never double dip*. Trust me, you can survive without having sex more than once a day. The only patients I've seen with priapism in years have been men who decided they knew more about dosing alprostadil than I did. They didn't, and their penises lived (barely) to regret it.

INTRAURETHRAL THERAPY: THE KINDER, GENTLER INJECTION

Not all males are as brave as Dr. Brindley. In order to deliver alprostadil without the prick, the Vivus Corporation developed a device called **MUSE (Medicated Urethral System for Erection)**. A plastic applicator the size of a matchstick is inserted about an inch into the urethra and squeezed to deliver a small (1 × 3–millimeter) semisolid alprostadil pellet (see Fig. 7). Theoretically, the medication is absorbed through the urethra into the erectile tissue and works just like ICP.

Why did we need MUSE? Its very existence shows that, although ICP works well, many men are scared of the needle. Why some men preferred inserting a plastic applicator into the urethra instead of a small needle into the shaft of the penis was never clear. Nevertheless, the release of MUSE was big news for those hoping to do away with the needle.

Urinating just prior to MUSE insertion makes the urethra more acidic, which helps dissolve the pellet. After inserting the pellet, you are instructed to hold the penis upright and stretched to its full length. The penis is then rubbed and rolled between the hands for about thirty to sixty seconds. Interestingly, almost 20 percent of men receiving a placebo (fake) pellet reported normal erections after doing all that pulling and rubbing.

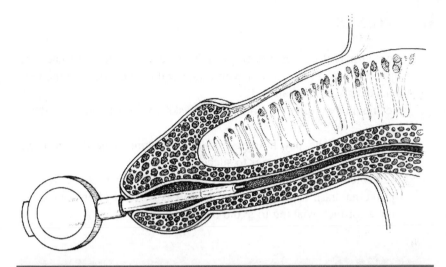

Fig. 7. Insertion of the stem of the MUSE applicator into the urethra.
(Illustration courtesy of the Vivus Corporation, Mountain View, California.)

The initial studies on MUSE showed decent success rates. However, when it gained FDA approval and was widely released, the number of patients responding favorably was less impressive. Success rates are less than half as high as for injection therapy. While only 10 percent of men using ICP complain of pain, about one-third of MUSE patients have. Since more of the vasodilator alprostadil is absorbed into the bloodstream, the first dose is often administered in the office to watch for fainting from low blood pressure.[1]

Although not applicable to large numbers of patients, the MUSE system continues to have a small following. Some of these are men especially apprehensive about needles (you know who you are). Blind men are also appropriate patients, since manually placing the applicator into the urethra is easier than properly placing a needle with impaired vision. Some men with psychogenic impotence also continue to use the MUSE. They probably get some response to the MUSE, but may actually benefit more from the confidence they gain.

One thing the Vivus Corporation clearly did do particularly well was the simultaneous development of the **Actis ring**, thee soft constriction ring meant to help hold the MUSE and the blood inside the corporal bodies. This is the best **constriction ring** available and can be used with or without MUSE for men with venous leakage (see chapters 11 and 15).

KEY POINTS

- Intracorporeal pharmacotherapy (ICP) offers an excellent treatment option for men that can't or won't take oral medications for the reasons discussed in chapter 12.
- Results are excellent as long as the risks are understood and dealt with.
- Overcoming the psychological idea of sticking a needle into the penis is the greatest barrier to success.
- Medicated Urethral System for Erection (MUSE) is a needle-free option that hasn't shown to work as well as ICP, but offers and alternative for men wishing to avoid the needle.

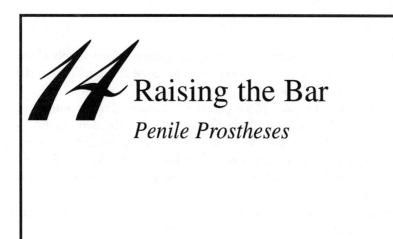

Raising the Bar
Penile Prostheses

Old truckers don't die. They just get another Peterbilt.

—Anonymous

*O*ne of the most motivated patients I ever met was Albert. Sex on a daily basis was his view of how life was supposed to be. He was one of the first men to take Viagra when it came on the market in 1998. It usually worked, but it wasn't capable of overcoming the naturally longer latency periods of a seventy-year-old smoker. He used a **vacuum constriction device** and tried **ICP**, but they never were satisfactory to him due to the lack of spontaneity. Once he came to this realization, he had to choose between less frequent intercourse and placement of a **penile prosthesis**.

Albert made the informed decision to have an inflatable penile prosthesis surgically placed. After a recovery period of about two months, when the penile swelling and tenderness resolved, he gave it a test drive. An immediate erection occurred with a few squeezes on the hidden pump. Thereafter, he was able to have an erection at will—limited only by his stamina (and that of his wife).

Despite the plethora of options discussed in the preceding chapters, some men will still not be adequately treated by nonsurgical intervention. They might not achieve an adequate erection or might not like the lack of spontaneity. Many men don't like the needle required for ICP. For their own reasons, they might just dislike the nonsurgical options. Albert simply chose the reliability of erection on demand. Whichever of these reasons is the case, surgery can be a godsend.

We can now surgically place penile prostheses—devices implanted inside the penis that stiffen it mechanically instead of through physiological processes. Although surgery is required, patient satisfaction is greater for those who receive penile prostheses than for any other form of therapy. Yes, greater than the satisfaction rates reported with Viagra and other oral medications.

Most prostheses are the inflatable type, using a hydraulic system to fill cylinders surgically implanted into the **corporal bodies**. When filled, they elevate the penis like normal erections. Some men prefer the older style **malleable** (otherwise known as **semirigid**) **prostheses**, which are simpler in that they have fewer or no moving parts. These noninflatable prostheses are also called *rod prostheses*, a particularly appropriate name.

EARLY PROSTHESES:
THE LONG, HARD ROAD TO SUCCESS

The introduction of penile prostheses is one of the great examples of medicine and industry working together to solve a complex problem. Ultimately successful, it was not a straight path to success. Investigators in 1936 implanted rib cartilage to stiffen the member. This worked in the short term, but the cartilage was degraded by natural body processes in a matter of months, leaving the patient even worse than before his operation. Not only did the penis not work, it was then full of spongy cartilage. That made it obvious a permanent material would be required.

The next step was the introduction of rigid rods that could be placed into the corporal bodies. They seldom failed, as the engineering required was as straightforward as the stiff rods, but the patients usually looked like sophomores embarrassed at the chalkboard. With no room for wiggle, they were often uncomfortable. If the least bit too long, they might erode out the end of the penis or into the **urethra** due to their unforgiving stiffness. No matter how you shifted the penis, it never fit well into Levis.

The next generation of prostheses was designed around a ratcheted core that could be "clicked" into position. They could be easily adjusted to whatever adventurous vertical angle a man was willing to try.

Semirigid or malleable (slightly bendable) prostheses followed. They could be put into any conceivable anatomical position. The Small-Carrion malleable prosthesis was named after the two surgeons who invented it. (No disrespect to Dr. Small, but that name should never be used with such a device.) Their initial sponge-filled device was soon replaced by options that incorporated a braided set of silver wires capable of multiple bends.

These semirigid devices were popular during the 1970s and 1980s, while silver prices were skyrocketing. Although the Hunt brothers of Texas were blamed for the precious metal's rise and fall in price, the silver used in these prostheses surely played some role in the madness. Unfortunately, no metal could stand the repeated rise and fall over the years, so eventually the wires sagged like the price of silver. The result is obvious. The semirigid prostheses became more *semi* than *rigid*.

The final step in this collaboration of medicine and industry occurred when Dr. Brantley Scott joined a biomedical engineer and a neurologist to form American Medical Systems (AMS) of Minnetonka, Minnesota. In 1973, they introduced the inflatable penile prosthesis (IPP). Three decades later, Dr. Scott's original design is still essentially intact in the IPPs used today. They are reliable and amazingly close to a normal-appearing erection.

MALLEABLE (ROD) PROSTHESES: FULL-TIME WORKERS

The simplest options are these noninflatable descendants of the early devices. They are straightforward to place surgically and hardly ever fail. However, they are not as popular due to the fact they supply a constantly firm penis. This can be hard to hide, even with loose pants on. These semirigid rods are "malleable," meaning they can be bent (but not broken, see Fig. 8). The *AMS 650, Mentor Malleable* and *Mentor Acu-Form* are the current versions available. *The Dura-II* is a slightly more sophisticated alternative, using a spring on each end of a central cable that allows the device to be placed in a greater number of positions.

PUMPED UP: HOW INFLATABLE PROSTHESES WORK

Most modern prostheses are based on hydraulic principles, where fluid from a reservoir is pumped into the two cylinders on demand. This fills the cylinders under pressure (sound like the normal erection?) until they stand

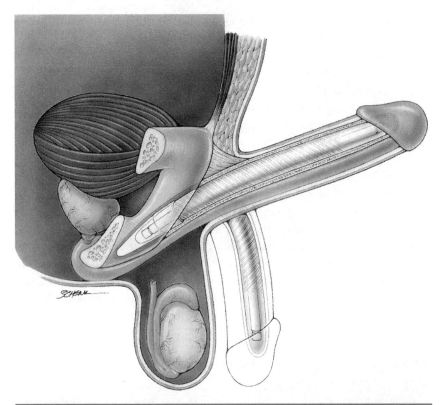

Fig. 8. Malleable (semirigid) prosthesis
shown in the active and neutral positions.
(Illustration courtesy of American Medical Systems, Inc.,
Minnetonka, Minnesota.)

erect. They come in *two-piece* and *three-piece versions*, each of which has its advocates. The terms *two-piece* and *three-piece* are both a little bit misleading, in that each has two cylinders that count as one. The differences are discussed below.

All the inflatable devices have a *reservoir* and a *pump*. The one-piece devices were the simplest ones to place surgically, but their success was not long-lived, and they are no longer available in the United States.

Two-piece devices come with all the components preconnected for simpler placement. The *AMS Ambicor* has a pump, implanted into the **scrotum** that forces fluid from the base of the prosthesis into the working end (see Fig. 9). The scrotal part is discreetly placed, slyly sitting in the

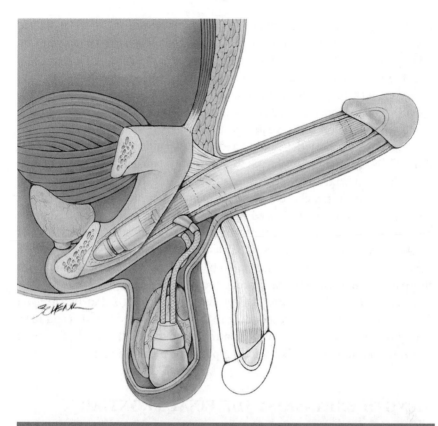

Fig. 9. Two-piece inflatable penile prosthesis (Ambicor).
(Illustration courtesy of American Medical Systems, Inc.,
Minnetonka, Minnesota.)

scrotum like a third testicle. They can be felt through the skin by a partner but are unnoticeable to the naked eye. This allows undressing in the locker room without fear of discovery.

Two-piece prostheses have stood the test of time. Many surgeons prefer these because of their relative ease in placement. Since everything comes preconnected, they are quickly placed and there is little chance of fluid leakage. They stiffen but don't expand much, so there is some sacrifice for the convenience of easier surgical placement. This is usually not an issue to the couple, so most patients end up happy. A good squeeze or two quickly fills the cylinders to full attention.

Three-piece devices—the gold standard—require more time and skill to place. They are softer when deflated, mimicking the normal flaccid penis. In the erect state, they are more rigid than the other versions, mimicking the normal erection. They require greater volumes of fluid in order to exhibit such a distinct difference in the erect and flaccid states, so a larger reservoir must be placed inside the abdomen. American Medical Systems (AMS) has the most experience with these devices, being the originator along with Dr. Scott thirty years ago.

The *AMS CX* provides rigidity and girth expansion. Its little brother, the *AMS CXM*, is essentially the same thing, only smaller. Originally, it was made for men with small penises (not the kind of thing a company advertises). It is most often chosen for use in men with scarred penises that won't allow placement of the full-sized models. Interestingly, it was created at the request of a group of Asian urologists, who claimed they needed smaller cylinders in their part of the world. True to the discussion in chapter 2 about penis size, their prejudice turned out to be incorrect, and many of the men in that part of the world who have penile prostheses use the standard implants.

The Mentor Corporation also produces the *Alpha I* and the *Alpha I Narrow Base*, roughly corresponding to the AMS CX and CXM. Their marketing department should have given more thought to the name; the word "narrow" doesn't sound like a selling point for penile implants.

LENGTH EXPANSION: THE FINAL FRONTIER

The final hurdle to cross for these devices was in length expansion. Until 1990, the prostheses could provide rigidity and girth expansion but could not expand in length due to engineering limitations. AMS then introduced its premier version, named wisely by their marketing department as the *AMS Ultrex* (see Fig. 10). The Ultrex is a direct descendant of Dr. Scott's original invention.

The original Ultrex was more prone to mechanical failure than other devices owing to the tricky structural needs of length expansion. This was corrected by strengthening the middle layer in 1993. Among all surgical and nonsurgical treatments, this is the closest we have come to a guaranteed, natural-looking erection.

Even so, it is crucial that men considering prosthesis surgery understand that no surgical correction can ever be as good as a normal natural erection. Although reliable to the highest degree currently possible, it is still man-made. The best inflatable penile prosthesis will never match the erec-

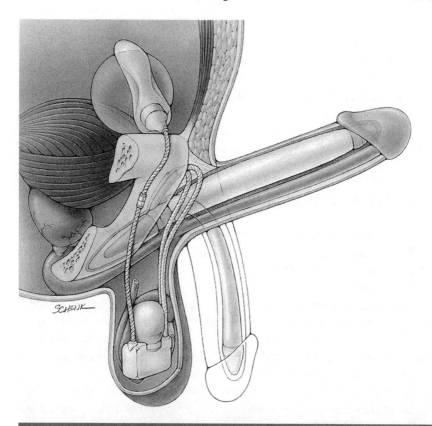

Fig. 10. Three-piece inflatable penile prosthesis (Ultrex).
(Illustration courtesy of American Medical Systems, Inc.,
Minnetonka, Minnesota.)

tions the patient had when things were perfect on their own. The main area surgery often doesn't meet expectations is in size. Even with the expansion provided by the newest devices, men often feel their penises don't stretch to their previous glory.

Part of this perception is real. The engineers have created masterpieces, but they can't work miracles. The laws of physics can't be broken, not even by the masters at these companies. In addition, men tend to have a selective memory when it comes to penis size. Remember, Masters and Johnson found out that men lie about the size of their penises. Well, maybe they just didn't remember the truth. When a man hasn't had a full erection for years, he sometimes revels in the glory of days past. He really didn't score the game-winning touchdown during his senior year homecoming game, nor did he really have that nine-inch monster he told his buddies about.

The penis is a balloon with a fixed length. Once inflated again—with a prosthesis this time instead of blood—it pretty much fills whatever space the balloon has. This balloon stretches to full, but can stretch no further. The nine-inch monster often turns out to be a four- to five-inch normal penis when reality sets in. A good reality check before surgery can prepare the patient for the ultimate reality that life—and anatomy—has dealt him.

WHICH PROSTHESIS IS BEST?

Frank and Ben were diabetic brothers who both had developed impotence. Frank underwent placement of an inflatable penile prosthesis and was very pleased with his results. Thereafter, he was always able to keep up with his younger wife.

When Ben heard of his little brother's success, he went to the same urologist to request an inflatable penile prosthesis. However, the older brother had severe rheumatoid arthritis that limited his manual dexterity. He was committed to having the prosthesis Frank had, but his finger agility was poor. With a demo model of the inflatable device on the examining room table, he had trouble compressing the pump that inflated the prosthesis. It was clear that there was no way he would be able to inflate and deflate it reliably if the device were within the scrotum.

Ben was disappointed, but not willing to give up. The rheumatoid arthritis could slow him down, but not keep him down. He chose to have a malleable prosthesis. Although he didn't have the fine motor skills to manipulate the small parts on the inflatable device, he was able to maneuver the malleable prosthesis into position whenever the opportunity arose.

There is no such thing as *the* best, but one version may be best for you. Each type should provide adequate rigidity when needed and should mimic the normal flaccid penis when not in use. The three-piece devices come closest to those goals, as their larger reservoir size allows there to be a greater difference between the full (rigid) and empty (flaccid) states.

Three primary considerations come into play:

- *Surgeon preference.* This is probably the most common reason a device is chosen. Surgeons develop comfort with what works well for them. If the doctor has many satisfied patients, he will probably be unlikely to argue with success until there is a strong reason to change.

- *Patient preference.* Some men may have a friend or a family member who has had a successful implant. They will hear the good things about that type and will want the same thing. Conversely, if a friend is dissatisfied with a particular implant, it is highly unlikely he will be open-minded. Some patients want the "Cadillac," but some prefer simplicity.
- *Cost.* These devices are very expensive. In addition, the fee for extra time in the operating room for implantation of the three-piece devices adds up. Even if insurance is paying for 80 percent of the cost, the other 20 percent of a several-thousand-dollar bill can be an issue. Without insurance, men may want the least expensive option that will meet their needs. Fortunately, insurers cover these operations well. If the primary insurance is Medicare, and if the patient has *secondary insurance,** there should be no out-of-pocket cost to the patient.

Our institution uses the AMS products due to their long history of innovation and reliability, but many physicians are pleased with their results using the other products mentioned above. The greatest length possibilities exist with the Ultrex due to its ability to increase in length during erection. However, it is not quite as stable as the more rigid AMS CX is, so some men with longer penises might prefer the latter.

CHOOSING A SURGEON

Choosing the right surgeon is crucial. Many patients spend more time choosing a cable company than choosing a surgeon. These operations require the skills of someone who understands the important details for success. Someone who performs the operations infrequently may not be as facile or up to date. He may be more likely to make small technical errors resulting in infection or device failure.

Following most operations, an infection may be only a minor setback, but an infected prosthesis will require a second operation to remove the

---

*Medicare covers 80 percent of all reasonable charges. *Secondary insurance* is a separate policy patients can (and should) purchase to cover the other 20 percent. These policies can be expensive, but most patients are wise to purchase them at the time they become eligible for Medicare and maintain them. After the initial eligibility period, patients have to qualify with a medical examination, so don't wait until you need the additional coverage. Otherwise, your health will probably keep you from affording the coverage you need.

device. Proper sizing of the cylinders requires skill that comes only with experience. Finally, the most complex prostheses require perfect connections between the parts to function properly. These connections are easy for surgeons with experience, but require ongoing familiarity to avoid the little pitfalls. In prosthesis surgery, the little details are crucial. Something as seemingly trivial as failure to get tiny air bubbles out of the tubing can affect fluid transfer and lead to failure.

For these reasons, we have two surgeons (Dr. Drogo K. Montague and Dr. Kenneth W. Angermeier) at the Cleveland Clinic Foundation Hospital who perform the majority of these operations. Patients benefit by knowing they have an experienced surgeon. The surgeons benefit by keeping their skills sharp.

This is not to say that only surgeons who specialize in these operations should perform all prosthesis surgery. Many fine general urologists do a great job on the operations—especially in smaller practices where they may truly be prosthetic surgeons who have to provide many other urological services based on their practice demographics.

The companies that make these devices keep lists of the surgeons who perform large numbers of prosthetic operations. Inclusion on these lists doesn't guarantee skill, but it is a good starting point for someone anticipating needing one.

DEVICES FOR SPECIAL SITUATIONS

Years of taking Vitamin E had failed to halt the progression of **Peyronie's disease**. Nathan found himself with an erection that bent back on itself more than ninety degrees. The curvature during the early years allowed vaginal penetration if he used enough lubrication, but no amount of KY jelly could overcome the doubled-over penis. He and his wife became so frustrated that they quit attempting intercourse.

Nathan started using the Internet during the late nineties and joined a chat room of Peyronie's disease patients. He learned that many of the members of the chat room had done well without surgery, but a small subset had undergone surgery to correct the curvature.

On examination, Nathan had a large plaque on the lower (ventral) aspect of his penile shaft. Since he was already impotent, it wouldn't help just to straighten out the organ. Therefore, he had surgery to place a dermal (skin) graft on the shortened side of the penis in order to straighten the organ and allow it to reach its natural length, followed by placement of a penile prosthesis.

It was felt that the extensive scarring from Peyronie's disease required one of the more rigid options. Nathan's surgeon placed an AMS CX, which gave enough rigidity for intercourse about eight weeks postoperatively. The Peyronie's plaque persisted after surgery, but the strength of the device allowed adequate, and straight, erections.

Some situations may indicate the need to choose one device over the others. Patients exhibiting severe scarring (including those with Peyronie's disease like Nathan) need the stiffness of a three-piece or a malleable prosthesis. Some elderly or disabled men with urinary troubles use an external catheter to collect urine into a bag when they can't void normally on their own. These catheters, sometimes called "Texas rigs," will sometimes stay on better if a malleable prosthesis holds the penis a little stiffer. This can be a double-edged sword, as these men also are prone to decreased sensation, so a prosthesis can erode its way out the end of the penis without the patient sensing anything wrong.

Men with long penises may prioritize the stability of an AMS CX over length expansion, whereas men concerned about small penis size will like the 1- to 2-centimeter extension of the Ultrex.

GETTING READY FOR SURGERY

As usual, there is good news and bad news. The good news is that prostheses usually work, and if they don't, they can be fixed. The bad news is, surgery is required. The incisions are small, but no man would call surgery on his penis "minor." Even if everything goes perfectly, the penis is tender and swollen for a few weeks, so action is out of the question until then. Fortunately, the swelling is all on the outside, so it doesn't interfere with urination.

In preparation for the operation, patients are often asked to shower in Hibiclens, Phisohex, or some other antimicrobial soap, especially in the groin area. This decreases bacteria that might infect the device. Antibiotics are given intravenously (into the IV tubing) right before the operation so that they can go directly into the bloodstream to kill any bacteria. Often, two or more antibiotics are used. That way, if bacteria are resistant to one antibiotic, the other should still prevent infection.

When in the operating room, the patient is placed under anesthesia. This can be done using either *general anesthesia*, where the patient is "completely out," or *regional anesthesia*. Regional anesthesia is usually by a *spinal block*, where a long needle is inserted through the skin of the back into the spinal column. There, a local anesthetic similar to those given by dentists is injected into the spinal fluid to block all the nerves going to the lower half of the body. Alternatively, an epidural catheter is a small tube (smaller than the size of a pencil lead) inserted into the spinal column where the nerves exit the canal. Through this tubing, anesthetic agents or narcotics can be administered continuously to block sensation. Since the duration of these operations is predictable, a single injection of a spinal block is usually easiest. The epidural can be re-dosed, however, if the operation lasts longer than usual or if the patient still experiences sensation following injection.

All the skin in the area is shaved immediately prior to the operation. Shaving earlier than that may cause small scratches in the skin that bacteria will grow into overnight and increase the bacterial count. The skin is then sterilized with a solution (often Betadine or Hibiclens) for up to ten minutes in order to kill as many bacteria as possible. While this is occurring, the members of the surgical team scrub their hands with similar solutions. Sterile surgical drapes (sheets) are then placed over everything except the actual operative site—in this case the lower abdomen and genitals. Sometimes even these areas are covered with a sticky sheet of clear plastic to seal off everything except the actual incision. The surgical team will wear sterile gowns and gloves as a final barrier to infection.

Due to the fear of infection, some surgeons even operate in specially designed rooms that circulate the air in a controlled fashion. Alternatively, there are air-filled devices that can be placed over the patient that essentially make the penis "the boy in the bubble." Like astronauts, the surgeon places his hands into sleeves extending inside the bubble, operating like scientists in "virus movies." These complex and expensive maneuvers have not been universally accepted, since there is no good proof they decrease the risk of infection.

CUTTING TO THE POINT

When all preparations are completed, the surgeon will make one or two incisions. The site and number depend on the device, the patient's anatomy, and surgeon preference.

The first option is an *infrapubic incision*, made just below the pubic bone where the top of the penis exits the body wall. This incision is used by some urologists because it allows them to easily place the reservoir into the lower abdomen. Due to the location of the incision, the urologist can see what he is doing while placing the reservoir instead of having to create a tunnel using his finger like he has to do if he uses the *penoscrotal incision* described below. The disadvantage is that it limits exposure to the root of the penis. Exposure for placement of a scrotal pump is also more difficult. Finally, the *dorsal penile nerve* is near that location. If the nerve is accidentally severed, the penis will have permanent loss of sensation—not too popular for the patient wishing to make his sex life better.

The other option is a *penoscrotal incision*, which is made either horizontally or vertically under the junction of the penis and scrotum. The penile nerve is protected, so penile sensation is not at risk. This incision allows the best exposure to the root of the penis, assuring the best placement of the cylinders and pump. The main disadvantage is that reservoir placement into the lower abdomen is more difficult if a three-piece device is chosen. A tunnel for reservoir placement can be created blindly by many surgeons, but some are more comfortable making a second small incision above the pubic bone. This is especially appropriate in men who have had lower abdominal surgery such as hernia repair. A major cause of erectile dysfunction is the operation **radical prostatectomy**, used to treat prostate cancer. These men will have scarring in the area as a result of their previous operation and should probably have a second incision made for reservoir placement.

PLACING THE DEVICE

Through either incision, the midsection of the penis (where it exits the body wall—remember that half of the penis is inside the body) is exposed. A small incision is then made in each corporal body. The corporal bodies are dilated and measured so the proper-sized cylinder can be placed. Sutures to close the corporal bodies are placed prior to putting the cylinders in, so that the expensive cylinders aren't punctured by the suture needles. Otherwise, once punctured, they are irreparable and must be replaced with a completely new implant. The pump is then positioned in a convenient location in the scrotum—either on the side of the dominant hand or in the wall separating the two halves of the scrotum, called the *septum*. Surgeons placing a two-piece device are then finished. The incisions are irrigated with antibiotic solution and closed with several layers of absorbable sutures.

When a three-piece device is placed, the reservoir is positioned either blindly or by making a separate incision. With a catheter through the urethra keeping the bladder empty, the surgeon develops a space behind the pubic bone to hold the reservoir. If the space created isn't large enough, it will squeeze on the reservoir. This causes **auto-inflation**, or a spontaneous erection of the cylinders based purely on excess pressure exerted on the reservoir.

The final step prior to antibiotic irrigation and closure is for the surgeon to bring the tubing that connects the pump, reservoir, and cylinders all together. A special crimping tool makes an easy, watertight connection. As long as all the air bubbles are out, the system usually remains intact and functions well for years to come.

AFTER THE OPERATION

After surgery, patients spend a couple of hours in the recovery room until anesthesia begins to wear off. Some surgeons will leave in a catheter to drain the bladder overnight, but many patients can be managed as outpatients. The penis is taped to the lower abdomen initially. The first trial of using the device is held off until all swelling and tenderness have subsided, usually around four to six weeks after the operation.

WHY NOT JUST PUT IN BIGGER CYLINDERS?

As discussed in chapter 2, penile size varies, so prostheses must accommodate this. They come in a few standard sizes and can also accept *rear tip extenders* for a tailored fit.

It sounds like a great idea just to stuff a larger cylinder into the corporal body you were born with. However, prostheses that are too long will just buckle and cause an "S-shaped deformity." If the prosthesis is too long for the sock it's inside of, it causes buckling into a serpentine shape. This diagnosis is too obvious. The oversized prosthesis puts constant pressure against each end of the sock. If this isn't corrected, the device may erode right out the end. If this occurs, it can still be replaced, but there is a greater risk of complications. Replacement with a smaller cylinder fixes the problem.

A prosthesis that is too short will leave the **glans penis** unsupported. This droop is called the "SST deformity" because of its resemblance to the downward slant of the Concorde jet's nose. This may be corrected by a little nip and tuck or by replacement with a longer cylinder several months later, when the problem becomes evident.

INTRAOPERATIVE PROBLEMS

As the surgeon stretches (dilates) the corporal bodies, the instruments occasionally rupture through the **tunica albuginea**. When this is a limited rupture, it may be repaired and not cause problems. If this injury goes into the urethra there is a high probability of infection, so the cylinder on this side is not placed. When this problem occurs, a tube might be left in the injured side to irrigate with antibiotics to lessen scarring and improve the chances a cylinder might be successfully placed a few weeks later, when things heal adequately.

The biggest fear of prosthetic surgeons is infection, occurring between 0.6 percent and 8.9 percent of the time.[1] The lower number is a reasonable expectation in good hands these days. Infection is usually due to microscopic bacteria sticking to the prosthesis. Even after all the sterile preparation and antibiotics described earlier, it is impossible to truly remove every single bacterium from the patient. It takes only a few of the little germs to settle on the implant and reproduce until an infection becomes evident. Diabetics are traditionally more susceptible to infection of the prosthesis, although it appears this is mainly in poorly controlled Type I (insulin-dependent) **diabetes**. Patients with spinal cord injuries are also more likely to have infections. Radiation treatments for prostate cancer were once thought to be a risk factor, but this is probably no longer true.

MAINTENANCE ISSUES

No mechanical device will ever be 100 percent foolproof. Indeed, these devices can break down and quit working. Due to their complexity, three-piece devices are more likely to fail, but this risk is often worth it in patients desiring a more natural-looking implant.

Most reports show the failure rate to be somewhere around 10 to 20 percent for most of these devices.[2] The fluid can leak out, resulting in inadequate pressure in the cylinders. The pump can fail. Although the lifespan of the Ultrex device was much less than that of other devices when first introduced, modifications to strengthen the weave of the middle fabric layer apparently have made a huge difference. A recent study from Drs.

Montague and Angermeier found that 94 percent of the improved Ultrex prostheses were still functioning properly after five years.[3] With any luck, they will last for as long as patients wishes to use them.

Infections are usually evident within the first three months. Pain, swelling, warmth, and sometimes drainage are the signs. Later infections occur when bacteria get into the bloodstream during dental work or other procedures. Less often, this can occur as a result of serious bacterial infections such as pneumonia. As these germs circulate by the prosthesis, it looks to them like a great place to setup house. They love to take up residence on any synthetic (man-made) material placed in the body. The synthetic material serves as a fort to protect the bacteria so they can set up an infection. Once infected, the bacteria are too protected for even the strongest antibiotics to kill. Their fortress—the prosthesis—must then be removed.

For this reason, people with any prosthetic device (anywhere in the body, not just in the penis) are often administered antibiotics during future surgical or dental procedures, or at other times when bacteria might get into the bloodstream. Then, the bacteria may be dead on arrival at the fort. In addition, AMS incorporates an antibiotic coating called *inhibizone* that helps prevent infection as well.

Until recently, it was felt that an infected prosthesis should be removed and not replaced until the patient had received a prolonged schedule of antibiotics to sterilize the area. However, it has recently been shown that the prostheses can frequently be replaced during the same operation and will usually be fine.[4]

SCARED OF SILICONE?

Based on the controversy surrounding breast implants, some men are concerned about silicone in these prostheses. They do contain silicone in their solid parts, but no modern prostheses contain silicone gel inside that could leak out.

REPLACEMENT

Unfortunately, there's never been a machine made that couldn't break down. If your carburetor dies, you can pull up the hood and tinker with it or replace it. If your prosthesis fails, it means another operation.

The second time around is even more complex. Any of the complications listed above occur at a higher rate during replacement. However, once a prosthesis has been placed, the erectile tissues are destroyed. Thereafter, there are no other good options for erections due to the permanent changes, so replacement is usually necessary.

Corporeal **fibrosis** is the biggest reason replacement surgery is more difficult. This scarring of the corporal bodies makes the tissues more difficult to work with surgically and leaves less room for the device. More than one incision may be needed to overcome these difficulties. Due to the less room in the corpora, many surgeons will use either the *AMS CXM* or *Mentor Alpha I Narrow Base*. If the scarring is too severe, penile size may be compromised even more than usual. Patients having replacements performed in the setting of severe corporeal fibrosis must understand these limitations. That doesn't mean prostheses aren't a good option. In fact, they are the best hope for patients with severe fibrosis. Nevertheless, even the best prosthetic surgery can't overcome severe fibrosis, so some patients will be disappointed if they don't have a realistic understanding of their underlying problems.

ARE YOU HAPPY NOW?

Since impotence treatment using a penile prosthesis requires greater effort on the part of the patient and surgeon, you would expect a satisfactory outcome or it wouldn't be worth it. Most patients think it is. Between 80 and 90 percent of men and their partners are satisfied with their choice and would do it over again.[5] This is the highest satisfaction rate for any form of treatment. To the surprise of many, these patients report higher satisfaction than even oral therapy.

The most common complaint is the feeling the prosthesis isn't as long as desired. As we discussed earlier, a longer device won't change the true length of the penis, so these men have to accept that it's not the prosthesis that's shorter than they would like, but rather their own anatomy.

THE AGING PROSTHESIS

The final issue with prostheses involves longevity. Theirs, not yours. At some point, many men no longer have the need or opportunity to use an erection.

Old age, ill health, or the loss of a partner may make the prosthesis unnecessary. You can discontinue any other form of therapy at any time just by stopping it, but a penile prosthesis will be there for life unless it is surgically removed. This usually doesn't cause any problem, so it will usually just sit there like an old soldier hoping for an assignment that may never come.

Albert, whose choice for a penile prosthesis was described at the beginning of this chapter, had six satisfactory years with his implant. His wife died at that time, leaving him alone for the first time in over fifty years. Faithful to the end, he hasn't used it since her death. He doesn't think he will ever begin seeing anyone else, but he is comforted to know it is in place if he ever decides to.

Do I HAVE TO TRY ALL THE NONSURGICAL OPTIONS FIRST?

Because surgery is the most complex option, some people feel it is an alternative only after *all* other treatments have failed. This is not a reasonable position. Surgery isn't "the last hope." It is a very acceptable treatment option that is known for patient satisfaction greater than that for *any* other form of therapy for erectile dysfunction, including medications. Therefore if you are not satisfied with the other options, it is acceptable to explore the possibility of penile prosthesis surgery with a respected urologist. Chapter 16 delves into the decision algorithm men go through while weighing impotence options.

KEY POINTS

- Modern penile prostheses offer the most reliable form of therapy for erectile dysfunction.
- Satisfaction rates for prostheses exceed those for *all* other treatment options.
- No mechanical device is failure-proof. A minority of patients will require a "tune-up" to keep their prostheses working throughout a normal man's lifetime.

𝒥5 Less Common Surgical Options

𝓑 efore penile prostheses had even been envisioned, urologists dreamed of a surgical cure for erectile dysfunction. The initial attempts were the testicular transplants described in chapter 1. The idea was to treat impotence indirectly by overcoming the low hormones that were believed at that time to be the only physical cause of erectile dysfunction. These methods fell by the wayside due to their poor results. Their demise would have been predictable had they known at the time that most erectile dysfunction is due to vascular disease and not insufficient hormones.

In 1902, J. S. Wooten claimed the first direct surgical cure. He stated that erectile dysfunction was due to a loss of penis tissue tonicity and could be corrected by tying off the *superficial dorsal vein* of the penis. This would theoretically increase that tone to an adequate level. When others failed to find the same success, Dr. G. F. Lydston at the University of Illinois reported six years later that the problem was due to inadequate surgery. He proclaimed that the surgeons who couldn't make it work were simply not tying off enough veins. In addition to the superficial dorsal vein, he went inside *Buck's fascia* to ligate (tie) the *deep dorsal vein* inside the corpora. He also went to great lengths to tie off all small accessory veins, claiming that failure was due to missing these small vessels.

Dr. O. S. Lowsley tightened the bulbocavernosus and ischiocavernosus muscles around the root of the penis in 1935. When this was done in conjunction with tying off the dorsal vein, a majority of patients reported normal erections. No one else, nonetheless, was able to duplicate these results, so we now know that the operations probably didn't really improve erections in most patients. Even so, occasional patients might benefit from the procedures in certain circumstances.[1]

ARTERIAL SURGERY: RESTORING THE FOUNTAIN OF YOUTH

> We don't always cure cancer, but then again, we don't cure diabetes, high blood pressure, or many other diseases either. The best we can hope for is to manage most diseases. If we can do that, we have been successful.
>
> —Bill Tranum, M.D., oncologist

Since an erection is nothing more than the penis filling and staying filled with blood, it was inevitable that surgery to improve the fountain that fills the penis would be attempted. Although usually disappointing, this approach in special circumstances makes sense. In fact, penile vascular surgery is actually the only true *cure* for erectile dysfunction due to physical causes. In all other situation, we can *manage* the disorder with the options discussed earlier in this book, but we don't actually cure it.

However, if a surgically correctable vascular abnormality is successfully operated upon, the patient may truly recover normal function permanently and require no further therapy. Note the stipulation on the impotence being "due to physical causes." Indeed, we can cure or overcome erectile dysfunction due primarily to mental causes if the issues are addressed properly.

Most patients with blocked arteries to the penis suffer from **arteriosclerosis**, a generalized hardening of multiple arteries throughout the bloodstream. Each hardened area narrows the stream and keeps blood flow out of the penis. That means bypassing one clogged segment will only bring blood flow to another clogged segment, so arterial flow isn't improved much. In contrast, sometimes there is an isolated (solitary) short area in the penile arteries that is obstructed. If so, a bypass operation can restore blood flow between normal blood vessels on either side of the narrowing. This will sometimes restore normal flow.

For these reasons, it is crucial that these operations be performed only on patients with isolated obstruction and otherwise normal circulation. Obstruction is suggested by either a **RigiScan** or a **Doppler ultrasound** image that indicates impaired penile blood flow (as described in chapter 7). The only way to tell if the decreased flow is due to an isolated narrowing is to perform **arteriography**. By placing a small catheter through the groin arteries, X rays (arteriograms) can be performed on the **pudendal arteries** in a manner similar to the way heart arteries are evaluated for blockage. When radiographic contrast (dye) is injected, the arteries on the X rays should look like a map of a river system. The injuries are usually noted as obvious narrowings. If there are multiple narrowings along these vessels then systemic arteriosclerosis can be diagnosed, which will negate the possibility of a bypass. However, a bypass might be an option if the rivers elsewhere look normal except for a solitary narrowing that is the only thing keeping blood out of the penis.

Arteriography should be reserved for younger patients with that have a reason to suspect this type of obstruction (see chapter 7). This suspicion might come from a history of pelvic fracture that could have disrupted an artery. These fine pudendal arteries can be trapped by the broken pelvic bones and thus rendered unable to supply the penis adequately.

A more common reason to suspect injury these days is when a man has a substantial history of bicycling. Bicycle seat pressure injuries occur when the rider puts too much pressure onto the pudendal arteries where they run inside the pelvic bones. These arteries are positioned under the pelvic bones in a manner that allows them to be compressed with this action. With prolonged time in the saddle, these arteries can become damaged and completely blocked. Prevention is key (see chapter 6). Once the damage has occurred, arteriography should be performed to determine if the obstruction is localized enough to be bypassed.

Revascularization operations work like a heart bypass. The obstructed area is bypassed by mobilizing the artery and bringing the two healthy ends together. If the obstructed part of the artery is too long to do that, sometimes a healthy vessel nearby (that doesn't supply a vital organ such as the penis) is used instead.

These operations require the surgeon to sew tiny arteries together with an opening between them large enough to stay open. The arteries are so tiny that the entire operation is performed using surgical microscopes.

Unfortunately, most arterial obstruction is due to diffuse arterial disease of arteriosclerosis. Bypass for these patients has proven essentially useless. These diseased arteries run all the way into the penis, so no bypass will overcome this resistance.

These operations are so uncommon that only a few centers around the country are prepared to do them properly. If such a lesion is suspected, your urologist will probably refer you to the nearest research hospital to consider repair.

VENOUS INSUFFICIENCY

Willie Johnson was a high school math teacher who never married. In his forties, there were rumors that he was gay, since no one had ever known of him to show interest in or to date women. However, he could more appropriately be described as appearing asexual. When Karen, a music teacher, tried to interest Willie in socializing he found an excuse to avoid the interactions. Despite his initial reticence, they soon began spending time together. Their first interactions were during school functions, but they both enjoyed each other's company enough that weekend dates followed.

Karen was pleased at first that Willie made no overtures. They fell in love and enjoyed each other in every way except sexually. After several months, Karen made it clear one night that his advances would be welcome. Willie feigned illness and said he should go home. Karen prepared a goody basket and brought it to Willie the following day. He didn't appear ill but seemed distant. Subsequent attempts to reestablish contact were unsuccessful.

Willie came to the office for an appointment that was scheduled to address "prostate problems." As discussed in chapter 9, this is often a euphemism for erectile dysfunction, so I asked Willie about his erections. "I can't get one," he admitted.

As we explored the severity and duration of the problem, a surprising revelation ensued. I asked the standard question, "When was the last time you were able to successfully achieve vaginal penetration?"

"Never," he replied.

This begged the question of Willie's sexual orientation, but he denied being homosexual as well. "I just haven't ever had sex," he explained.

Although uncommon, some men reach Willie's age without sexual activity. The most common reason is for moral or religious reasons prohibiting premarital intercourse. He denied that the problem was morally based. "I've never been able to have an erection, doc!" he blurted out. "Not in the morning. Not with masturbation. And definitely not with a woman!"

More men have venous leakage than are usually recognized. These men don't have enough outflow resistance to allow blood to become trapped inside the penis under adequate pressure. Some of them will initially get an erection, but it goes down again easily, especially during pelvic thrusting.

Utilizing the same **constriction ring** that is used with a **VCD** can give excellent results slowing outflow just enough to make all the difference. Men with mild **venous insufficiency** may also respond to pelvic floor muscle exercises. This is best done under the direction of a physiotherapist who supervises an active program. However, treatment is intense, expensive, and often unsuccessful, so it will not be a reasonable option for most men.

Common sense implies that tying off some of the more than adequate veins draining the penis would improve erections in these patients. Surgeons of the early twentieth century worked long and hard to make the concept work. Although initial reports drew rave reviews, it has become clear that these operations rarely provide long-term improvement. The reason that **venous ligation surgery** is usually not helpful relates to the fact that venous insufficiency is rarely due to just one or two easily identifiable veins that can be tied off. Instead, most men experiencing venous leakage have abnormal corporeal smooth muscle pathology (the muscles in their **sinusoids** are worn out and don't work, so they allow venous blood to flow out too easily) and not just a single, large, open vein.

Two situations may involve a large open vein amenable to surgical correction. The first is in a man who has primary impotence—in other words, he has never had the ability to maintain an adequate erection. He could have been born with a large open vein that allows a quick exit of blood flow from the penis. The second situation involves a man who has had injury to a vein from pelvic trauma, which might have even torn a hole in the **tunica albuginea.** Surgical correction might be a curative option in that setting.

As it turns out, Willie Johnson had suffered a pelvic fracture as a child during a motor vehicle accident. Further investigation, involving **cavernosography**, identified a large vein allowing blood to flow straight out of the **corporal bodies** as soon as it flowed in. He had primary impotence—he had *never* been able to have an erection—due to venous insufficiency. He was one of the rare patients that was a good candidate for venous ligation surgery.

SWELL! COMPLICATIONS OF PENILE VASCULAR SURGERY

If you think the penis swells up during an erection, you should see what happens following vascular surgery. Things really swell up for the first two or three weeks following the operation. This involves not only the penis, but the loose tissue in the **scrotum** as well. A small drainage tube may be placed under the skin of the penis and scrotum for a day or two in an effort to limit this. Ice packs help, but only so much.

Swelling of the glans penis occurs if the surgeon misses a communicating venous branch, which leads to even higher pressure. A return to surgery to tie off the offending branch will take care of the problem. Because the vessels being sewn are so small, the suture line can be disrupted and the vessels torn apart even with normal activities. This will lead to failure.

Up to 20 percent of patients will experience penile shortening and numbness from scar entrapment. As the scar tissue softens, sensation usually returns in twelve to eighteen months if no major nerve has been cut. If anything major has been cut, it may remain numb permanently. Therefore, these procedures should be done at a research center specializing in such complex operations, if at all.

SUCCESS WITH PENILE VASCULAR SURGERY

Recall that reports of vascular surgery indicated phenomenal success rates in the early twentieth century. The fact that you don't know of anyone who has had one of these operations attests to the fact that they haven't stood the test of time. In properly selected patients, it is expected that about 50 to 60 percent of these complex operations will result in return of erections. Venous surgery has been even less likely to succeed than arterial bypass.

Since a completely normal vascular system (other than the isolated lesion) is needed for the vascular penile operation to be successful, candidates should be selected very carefully. Men with insulin-dependent (Type I) **diabetes** develop such significant diffuse *microvascular disease* that they are ruled out almost automatically. Microvascular disease is defined as the selective narrowing of the smaller arteries in the body. Since the pudendal and penile arteries are small arteries, they are affected fairly early in the process. This is the main reason patients with Type I diabetes almost invariably develop erectile dysfunction as well as the reason they aren't candidates for penile revascularization (although they are good candidates for all the other treatment options).

Men who smoke also develop diffuse arterial disease. For this reason, most surgeons will not consider arterial bypass surgery on anyone still smoking. This is not discrimination; it is simply a realistic view of a patient's prognosis. It is hard to justify an expensive, risky bypass operation to restore blood flow to the penis in someone who is trying as hard as he can to reobstruct the artery.

Men who might be candidates and who stand the greatest chance of success with these uncommon operations are those who are otherwise healthy, but have a solitary area of obstruction. If they are willing to undergo a complex reconstruction, they might be cured.

KEY POINTS

- Penile vascular surgery is useful only in a rare patient with a solitary narrowing or obstruction of a vessel to the penis or a large abnormal vein allowing blood to run out of the penis unimpeded.
- These are unusual findings, so few patients will be candidates for penile revascularization or venous ligation surgery.
- The only *cure* for erectile dysfunction due to physical causes is possible only for the rare patient for whom vascular surgery is appropriate.

16 Choices, Choices
How Do I Decide?

What, therefore, cannot be cured, must be endured.
—Tobias George Smollett,
The Expedition of Humphry Clinker, 1771

*P*eople like simple answers. Before oral medications became available, the management of erectile dysfunction was difficult. First, men wanted to know why they had problems. Despite the biases of medicine through the years that impotence was psychogenic in origin, most men knew there was more to it than that. Therefore they wanted to find out why they couldn't get an erection. If they could only know why it happened, they reasoned, they could reverse the cause.

However, it was never that easy. Sure, it was occasionally obvious such as in cases where surgery had cut a nerve. However, recall that there are usually multiple issues causing erectile dysfunction in any given man. In chapter 6, Edward wanted to know whether his erectile dysfunction was due to smoking, diabetes, hypertension (high blood pressure), alcohol, medications, his weight, age, or sleep apnea. He was even willing to consider the possibility that the stresses between him and his wife could be the cause, or that job and financial pressures were taking their toll. In short, he wanted to know which one caused the problem. Unfortunately for Edward, it was all of them.

The major problem facing Edward was finding out that the cause was *multifactorial*—a combination of all these issues. The result was that even if he could change one, two, or eight of these concerns, he still had reasons remaining that could prevent his recovery unless he received treatment.

When multiple issues are present, some will inevitably be reversible and some will not. Edward was able to change a few things, such as his weight, blood pressure medication, and general health. He could manage his diabetes and hypertension, but they couldn't be cured. In fact, the medications to manage his hypertension actually contributed to his erectile dysfunction. He could stop smoking and drink responsibly. But he still couldn't make himself younger.

Before oral medication was available, the discussion with a urologist would center around changing as many issues as we could. However, men generally didn't like that option. In an age when people were used to going into the doctor's office with a problem and walking out with a prescription that would fix it, no man with erectile dysfunction liked what he was being told. No matter what the cause, men couldn't walk into the doctor's office and leave with a prescription that would magically cure all ills. These were the dark ages of erectile dysfunction.

PFIZER TO THE RESCUE

The introduction of **vacuum constriction devices** (see chapter 11, "The penis in a vacuum") and **intracorporeal injection** therapy (chapter 13) seems like ancient history, although they actually occurred in the waning years of the twentieth century. They provided two new options that allowed men to regain erections without surgery. Unfortunately, they were still more intricate than walking into the drugstore with a prescription and out with a magic pill, so men didn't beat the doors down. Therefore men still went to the doctor only when desperate for treatment.

The introduction of Viagra brought about a sea change in this thought process. Whereas erectile dysfunction treatments were complex prior to that time, men could suddenly ask for a prescription and take a pill later that night. It was as simple as treating a headache.

The number of men with erectile dysfunction didn't change on that day in 1998 when Viagra was released, but the number of diagnoses given in doctors' offices around the world sure did. Significantly, most men were treated for erectile dysfunction by urologists prior to that time. That changed immediately. Currently, 86 percent of Viagra prescriptions are written by nonurologists according to Pfizer. Most are written by primary care providers. There are around ten thousand urologists in North America, but six hundred thousand different physicians worldwide have written Viagra prescriptions. Nine Viagra tablets are prescribed every second—that's a lot of pills. Sixteen million men have taken the medication. Things have changed.

WHAT SHOULD I DO THE FIRST TIME I NOTICE A PROBLEM?

> Don't knock rationalization. Where would we be without it? I don't know anyone who'd get through the day without two or three juicy rationalizations. They're more important than sex. Have you ever gone a week without a rationalization?
> —Michael (Jeff Goldblum) in *The Big Chill*, 1983

Erectile dysfunction usually comes about slowly—insidiously—until something makes the man or woman suddenly aware of the issue. The decreased rigidity of the penis is usually noticed first by the man. A woman may not be able to tell the difference as long as the penis is erect enough for penetration. Vaginal stimulation might not change with firmness. This is based on the fact that vaginal stimulation is present only in the outer one-third of the **vagina**. Deeper than that, there may be some sensation of fullness, but this is not usually noticeable in the setting of significant stimulation elsewhere. It's like the concept that the splinter in your thumb won't bother you right after you stub your toe. The brain can receive only so much sensation at any given time and thus filters out much of the rest as background noise.

The astute man usually notices slight decreased rigidity. Often, this is perceived as a result of taking more time and effort to become fully erect. He probably didn't watch this process closely prior to that time, but suddenly he becomes concerned. Many men have confirmed the difference through masturbation prior to seeking help.

This may just be a nuisance for the relaxed couple, for when it doesn't require any changes as long as penetration continues to be possible. As you know by now, relaxing is not the natural reaction to a penis that's not as impressive as it used to be: panic sets in easily. A minor problem becomes a family crisis in a large number of cases.

For those who don't panic, this is the time to reassess your general health. Take a hint from the penis that there may be issues that should be addressed. If you haven't listened to any of the better reasons (like death), use this one to quit smoking. Now. Start eating better and get back into shape. If you are drinking more than two alcoholic drinks a day, cut back to this level or stop drinking altogether. Drinking to improve your sex life is like smoking to breathe better. If you can't walk straight under the influence, doesn't it make sense the penis won't be straight either? Any recreational drugs should be discontinued (and obviously shouldn't be used in the first place).

In short—it's time to realize you're a grown-up.

These lifestyle changes won't have an overnight effect. For most people, the problem didn't start just last night. Many of the underlying causes have arisen gradually in the years preceding the onset of impotence. Therefore, restoring perfect health overnight may not always be feasible. More importantly, we can't change some things about a patient's overall health. Chronic diseases like diabetes, hypertension, or **arteriosclerosis** take years to develop. Waking up one morning with a decision to be healthy won't work miracles, but if you put in the effort and are patient, rewards are possible.

Most men will be more likely to do anything but relax. They are likely to develop **performance anxiety** as discussed in chapter 10 (in the section titled, "The mind: it's a terrible thing to waste on sex"). Take a realistic look at your mental status. Are you stressed, anxious, or depressed? If so, is it you, or just your response to weakening erections? If it is innate, psychological help should be obtained. If it's performance anxiety, try not to worry! (See chapter 10 for a discussion of ways to avoid that trap.) If you're not sure, ask for appropriate help. This could be in the form of your primary care physician or a psychotherapist.

WHEN YOU FINALLY TALK TO THE DOCTOR

There is nothing wrong with making the positive nonmedical lifestyle changes described above, but don't feel that you have to wait to discuss the sexual issue with your physician. The most important reason to begin the discussion early is that the penis may be serving as a monitor of systemic health. As discussed in chapter 6 (in the section titled, "No penis is an island"), the same deterioration in health that you are noticing in the penis may be going on in the rest of your body. If this is the first sign of high blood pressure, arteriosclerosis, diabetes, or other serious health concern, the penis may bring it to your attention in time to save your life.

Consider with your physician whether any prescription medications are contributing to the problem. As discussed earlier, medications are often accused but rarely guilty. However, if you take a prescription medication known to frequently lead to erectile dysfunction, you could consider alternative medications with the prescribing physician. The most likely culprits include beta-blockers (e.g. propranolol), centrally acting antihypertensives (Aldomet and Clonidine), or psychoactive medications for depression, anxiety, sleep, or psychosis. Rarer causes are medications like estrogen, ketoconazole, and prostate cancer treatments that block **testosterone**.

Patients suspecting impotence from antidepressants theoretically might benefit from switching to *trazadone*. This antidepressant actually seems to increase erections and has been noted in the development of prolonged erections (see chapter 12, "Treating depression and erectile dysfunction"). Although the idea makes a lot of sense, it is usually better to make sure that the depression is treated optimally with whichever antidepressant works best and treat the erectile dysfunction separately. Trazadone is not as effective as SSRI medication as an antidepressant in most patients.

IF THE SIMPLE THINGS DON'T WORK

When the simple things don't work, make certain you go to the doctor if you haven't already done so. Ideally, you already have a primary care physician available to help with the problem. If you're old enough to be having difficulties, you're old enough to have a primary care physician. This person should be a professional that can help with most health needs, or refer you to a specialist if he isn't prepared to deal with any given issue. For most health problems, this would usually mean he would prefer that you have the benefit of expertise. For sexual problems, it may mean that he isn't comfortable with such personal issues. There is nothing wrong with that; we're all human, and some of us are more comfortable discussing sexual issues than others. It is better that the physician recognizes this than to stammer, stutter, and then not address the problem adequately. If he realizes that he isn't comfortable in dealing with sexual issues, he can make a referral to a urologist or someone else who is.

The primary care physician also doesn't have to be someone you'd socialize with, but it should be someone with whom you are comfortable. With the exception of significant personal feelings on your part, you should avoid choosing a physician based on gender. All physicians take the same classes.

BREAKING THE ICE

Dr. Kohler addressed multiple health issues during Jeff's annual physical examination. The blood pressure and cholesterol were slightly elevated. Both could be managed through diet and exercise, but the patient was taking neither seriously. Since Jeff was fifty years old, a colonoscopy was indicated to screen for colon cancer. Several blood tests were order, including a **prostate specific antigen (PSA)** test to check for prostate cancer. During the rectal examination, the doctor asked if Jeff was having any problems with urinary symptoms or erections. "They're both a little slower," Jeff conceded, facing away from the doctor due to the examination being performed.

Jeff's mild heart murmur and a few freckles were checked closely. Neither appeared to have worsened since last year. He wasn't perfect, but it seemed reasonable to Dr. Kohler that Jeff's health would be okay for another year.

"Anything else we should address while you're here?" the doctor asked with his hand already on the outer doorknob.

"Not really," Jeff answered as he tucked in his shirt.

That night Jeff failed yet once more to maintain an erection. His wife tried to be understanding, but she was frustrated when he told her the doctor didn't have any idea why he couldn't maintain an erection. "He checked my prostate and said it was fine. My cholesterol is a little high, though. That must be the problem." He didn't disclose that the doctor didn't find out why Jeff was impotent because Jeff failed to pursue the doctor's query.

"Did he offer you a sample pack to try?"

"No. I guess I'm not a good candidate because I have a heart murmur," he reasoned. "I'll ask him about an implant if it gets bad enough."

If you are the typical man with erectile dysfunction, the problem is about the only thing on your mind. There are no other issues in the world that approach the importance of assuring your penis recovers its lost youth. However, the rest of the world, with the exception of your mate, may be oblivious to your plight.

During a checkup, your physician will be assessing you for a number of problems. He is concerned with your blood pressure, with your general health, and with remembering whether you have had all the things recommended for routine health maintenance appropriate for your age. During your discussion, he may be checking your chart to make sure he has remembered to recommend a colonoscopy if you're over fifty. He may also be reviewing your medications to make sure your blood pressure pill won't interact with the new cholesterol medicine he is considering. He will probably be thinking of several other medical issues during your visit that he may not even mention to you because he's efficient at multitasking. He is also concerned with the numerous other patients he will see that day, in addition to the hospital staff meeting agenda for tonight. *You may have to bring up the subject.*

A good physician will regard this concern with as much seriousness as if you complained about an ache or pain. He will realize you are not just making small talk. He will realize you are reaching out for help with a health issue that is as important to you as diabetes or a broken foot.

If he doesn't pick up on your overture, make sure you were assertive enough in stating your concerns. If you mention it under your breath in a dismissive tone, as Jeff did, he may interpret that as your indication to him that you really aren't bothered by it or don't want to address it. Productive conversation requires that both parties contribute and listen, so you have some responsibility too. As it turns out, Jeff was experiencing mild erectile dysfunction. He was an excellent candidate to try **phosphodiesterase (PDE) inhibitors**. Had he simply made it clear that he considered the erections to be a problem, he could have had relief before nightfall. Instead, he had to wait until his next annual checkup to address the issue unless he was willing to make an appointment specifically to cover erectile dysfunction. You could guess that, if he wasn't able to discuss it openly during a face-to-face visit, he wasn't likely to take the initiative to schedule a second separate appointment to discuss the problem. He was this close to success yet failed to make it happen.

Despite assertive incursions into sexual issues, some physicians will either be too busy or simply unwilling to get involved in such personal matters. If your physician still doesn't address your concern when appropriately notified, it may be time to consider asking for a referral to a specialist or changing doctors.

None of this is to imply that the patient is responsible for communication instead of the doctor. On the contrary, we share the responsibility. The only difference is that if no one makes sure that the communication is received, you are the one whose needs aren't met.

WHAT ABOUT INTERNET TREATMENT?

> This trivial and vulgar way of union: it is the foolishest act a wise man commits in all his life. . . . What an odd and unworthy piece of folly he hath committed.
>
> —Thomas Browne, *Religio Medici*, 1643

The Internet has irrevocably changed our world. From the comfort of home we can obtain sports scores, help our children research a term paper on Celtic history, or trade stocks. It was only a matter of time before medical care became available on the Internet. Watch out. There is no accountability for the information presented, so anyone with a laptop can make any claims. More dangerously, you can buy vacuum constriction devices, constriction rings, injectables, or prescription medications such as Viagra simply by checking a few boxes on a Web site whose company is based in some unknown land.

Recall that in 1999 the *First International Consultation on Erectile Dysfunction* convened in Paris to review all the scientific information available on erectile dysfunction. Cosponsored by the World Health Organization (WHO) and *Société International d'Urologie*, they emphasized that medical treatments require the direct involvement of a physician and condemned Internet prescribing.

Although some consumers have expressed the opinion that these recommendations come from physicians' needs to "protect turf," this is not true. First, the WHO is far more motivated to assure access to quality care for underserved populations than it is to protect the salary of doctors in the United States. They couldn't care less if physician waiting rooms were empty in Cleveland, but they do care that patients are safely cared for throughout the world.

The second reason that this is not true relates to the need of each patient to have a physician looking closely at his individual situation concerning health care. As emphasized earlier, the penis is in some ways just a monitor of the rest of the patient's health. Therefore erectile dysfunction may be a sign of serious or life-threatening disease. These won't be detected by a Web site. In addition, although impotence treatments are usually safe, side effects are always a possibility. The Web site won't be there in the middle of the night if a problem should arise, and they sure won't be there to help you decide what to do if the treatment you got at the Web site doesn't meet your needs.

Recall that treatments as varied as a vacuum constriction device, injectables, and oral medications have been shown to have poor success rates without proper education but excellent success rates when proper instructions are given. The Web site won't care about how you use the products, as long as your credit card authorization comes through. Make an appointment with a physician you can trust. If you don't have one, let this be the time you change that.

THE GOAL-ORIENTED APPROACH

Once the doctor and patient agree on the diagnosis of erectile dysfunction, the patient is a candidate for the **goal-oriented approach** (assuming there are no serious systemic diseases to deal with first). Through this approach, instead of focusing on diagnostic tests to decide where the problem is, the focus is on *overcoming* the problem. It is based on the reality that treatment options are the same regardless of cause unless there is an obvious, readily reversible condition at the root of the problem. Since there are multifactorial issues at work most of the time, we don't try to zero in on the most important one but rather offer treatment that will overcome an array of causes.

Usually, the physician will ask a few questions such as those listed in chapter 7 (in the section titled, "Talking to the physician"). A *sexual health inventory* can quantify the degree of erectile dysfunction. These aren't absolutely necessary, but they help numerically validate the problem. This number can help some men understand it's not an insignificant problem and that treatment is justified.

This conversation is the cornerstone of management, so as soon as a few questions are covered, it is reasonable to move on to treatment. Any treatment can be offered at this point, but a trial of oral medication is usually initially considered based on its simplicity. The PDE inhibitors are the first and most successful medications as this book goes to print. Many times the medication gives patients enough satisfaction and confidence that they need no other therapy. If that is the case, the medication can be discontinued as soon as confidence returns. If not, the medications may be used as long as needed.

There are relatively few downsides to a trial of PDE inhibitors. They are very safe if you are healthy and are not taking nitroglycerin. Their side effects are usually reversible and not serious. In fact, most men who experience side effects still want to continue treatment because the medication worked. Men sometimes report a mild headache, but in their words, "it's worth it." Most other side effects are tolerable and unlikely to cause cessation of the medication.

The most common reason men fail to respond to PDE inhibitors is that they haven't taken them properly. The most common error is in taking an inadequate dose. Many primary care physicians are comfortable with prescribing 50 milligrams of Viagra, since that is the dose in the free sample packs. However, this dose may not be enough for men with more significant problems. Large men should also be offered the higher accepted doses before giving up. Fifty milligrams circulating through a 140-pound body will be much more concentrated in the penis than it will be if the dose is spread out over a 300-pound body.

Some men don't realize that these drugs work only by allowing the erection cycle to function normally. Their real role isn't in creating an erection—it is actually in keeping the arteries open once the process starts. Therefore, without sexual stimulation, the penis may be unmoved. Only with stimulation—sometimes surprisingly little—will the phosphodiesterase inhibitor exhibit activity. When that happens, a little penile rumbling that normally would have gone unnoticed may perk up and make its intent known.

CONSIDERING OTHER OPTIONS

Sometimes medications don't have their desired effect. If you are still having a problem after four or five serious attempts at taking oral medications, this is the point where you may want to seek the help of a urologist if you haven't already done so. Measurement of serum testosterone should be considered, especially if there is a decreased **libido**, or lack of interest in sex. Other blood tests may also be obtained if there is suspicion of hormonal abnormalities. Blood sugar levels, blood pressure, or other tests may be performed if the primary care physician hasn't already done so.

In occasional cases, further diagnostic tests may be considered (see chapter 7). In the spirit of the goal-oriented approach, they are used only if a vascular or other unusual injury is suspected, or if the man feels an intense "need to know." Otherwise, the same options will be available no matter what the tests show, so we move on to more involved treatments.

Like most other things in life, there are trade-offs with the more involved options offered by the urologist. The vacuum constriction device (VCD) (see chapter 11) is safest, as long as you don't let any adjacent parts get pulled inside the cylinder. It may be the only therapy known to man that has never had a death reported. Although the initial payment may be a few hundred dollars, it is virtually indestructible and may last a lifetime. Most insurance plans such as Medicare cover part or all of the cost. Because of the "fidget factor" (i.e., they take some work to create an erection), VCDs are usually most satisfactory in long-term relationships where both partners are willing to put in the effort.

A constriction ring can be used by itself without a VCD. When erectile dysfunction is mainly experienced as a good erection that goes down (detumesces) without **ejaculation**, these rings can slow down the exit of blood from the penis and keep things going without major cost or risk.

Intracorporeal pharmacotherapy (ICP) is even more successful than using a VCD (see chapter 13). Once injected, the erection looks natural. This is an advantage for a man who doesn't want to acknowledge he requires assistance in obtaining an erection. Many single men can excuse themselves to the restroom and inject in a matter of seconds. A partner will assume he's just emptying his bladder. When he returns and the action starts, she will never know it's not her charms that brought him to attention.

The worst aspect about ICP is the fact that most men don't like the idea of putting a needle into their penis. This is more of a mental block than anything, so most patients overcome this concern. The minimal discomfort is usually worth the outcome. If pain is an issue, most patients will have less discomfort if they try a different medication. Cost is an issue, at $3 to $35 per occasion. This adds up quickly if used on a regular basis. Scarring (**fibrosis**) and curvature are rare but must be considered in your decision. **Priapism** is rare with the newer medications but quite serious when it actually occurs.

Most men will try at least one, if not all, of the above treatments before seriously considering placement of a **penile prosthesis**. This doesn't mean they have to try all the options. Some physicians make their patients "walk the trail" from medications to vacuum devices to penile injections to surgery. It isn't necessary for the patient to try them all, as long as he has truly considered each option and made an informed decision on each. Some or all the other options may be contraindicated, or the patient may just not be willing to use certain options based on his own personal reasons. As long as his decision is fully informed (and not just because the doctor recommended surgery right off the bat), a penile prosthesis is a very reasonable option.

The advantage of a **penile prosthesis** is impressive in that almost anyone capable of withstanding an operation can regain erections. Recall that the erectile tissue is replaced by prostheses surgery, so there is no going back. That means you should make sure that this is the only option that is satisfactory to you before making a commitment.

On the other hand, don't let the permanence keep you from having a penile prosthesis if this is the right option for you. When men make the decision to have surgery, their satisfaction scores outpace that of any other treatment, including oral medications.

SHOULD MY ERECTIONS BE TESTED FIRST?

Recall that there are really two clinical indications for impotence testing to be performed beyond a history, physical examination, and cursory laboratory blood studies. These history, physical exam, and blood tests confirm that the patient is healthy enough to have sex and that no serious problems are in the way. The only absolute indication for further testing is when a man is considering vascular surgery (see chapter 15). These operations are occasionally indicated, but only when unequivocal proof is available that the underlying problem is surgically correctable.

The other group of men who are sometimes tested are those who "just have to know." Sometimes he is a bit egotistical, convinced that only some strange, inconceivable abnormality could explain his problem. He reasons that the physician just hasn't figured out the cause, so further tests will solve the mystery.

On the other hand, in some cases the physician believes erectile dysfunction is due to performance anxiety while the man is convinced he is physically incapable of having an erection. He denies that morning erections occur. There has to be a blockage!

The simplest tests to determine if the penis is capable of achieving an erection involve **nocturnal penile tumescence (NPT)** testing. The patient may try the **stamp test** at home. This will show if the penis ruptures a coil of stamps wrapped around its base during sleep. Or, a **snap gauge** can document the deed. This visible proof is usually all that is needed.

If these tests don't give a clear indication of penile blood flow (the snap gauge or the stamps show only a partial nocturnal erection), formal NPT testing is an option. The easiest way to do this is by a **RigiScan** performed over a three-night period at home. The device can be returned for interpretation as easily as returning a video rental. The only time a formal sleep lab study is required is when other problems such as **obstructive sleep apnea** are concurrently being assessed. Otherwise, this expensive and complex investigation gives little more information about erections than the RigiScan does. The other tests discussed in chapter 7 are used so rarely, they don't play a role in the standard patient being treated using the goal-oriented approach.

One should question the utility of testing altogether for most patients. Using the goal-oriented approach, diagnostic tests help only when the goal is to have a definitive answer. Otherwise, they almost always leave the patient with the same options regarding treatment. Therefore, if the treatment option is acceptable to the patient and he responds to it, nothing else is necessary.

When the RigiScan indicates severe arterial obstruction or venous leakage, the more involved studies may be indicated to see if vascular surgery would help. As discussed, it usually won't.

COST

Calculating the cost of medical care is trickier than it would appear. This is because cost depends on your perspective. Payment is usually made by a combination of the patient and his insurance company. Therefore the cost to the insurance company may be huge, but the patient may not care as long as his out-of-pocket expense is reasonable. On the other hand, the patient will care about every dime he is paying when he is footing the entire bill with no insurance coverage.

No one questions the need for health insurance to cover a heart attack or stroke, but in the past, some "lifestyle" issues such as erectile dysfunction have been considered frivolous and therefore not covered. The reasoning was that people die of heart attacks and serious diseases, but no one ever died of erectile dysfunction (although some have thought they would). This was unreasonable, of course. No one dies of a broken arm either, but an insurance company would never consider telling you to live with it. Fortunately, almost all insurers have abandoned this bias and have been good about covering erectile dysfunction as well as they cover other health issues.

Once insurance is in the equation, however, everyone has his own perspective on cost. The patient wants the best option available at the least cost to him. The insurer wants whatever keeps its responsibility the lowest. Finally, the physician wants a satisfied patient but also must make a living. These interests sometimes collide.

A good example of this concept involves a man in his early sixties with erectile dysfunction. He may respond adequately to oral medications. His insurance pays for six tablets a month, which is about half as many as he uses. If it is worth it to the patient, he can pay for the remainder out of pocket. He might alternatively decide that the extra cost is not worth it to him, so he would prefer to have a penile prosthesis placed. As it turns out, his hospitalization coverage is 100 percent, so he might have no out-of-pocket expense for the operation, compared to an ongoing expense of sixty dollars or more a month for the extra oral medication.

When this man reaches sixty-six years old—three years from now—the equation will change as he goes on Medicare. He will lose the prescription drug coverage that pays for some of his oral medications. Moreover, his Medicare will cover only 80 percent of the cost of his penile prosthesis if he waits until then. He can purchase a supplemental policy that will cover the extra 20 percent, but that ongoing monthly cost will be high and might keep him from doing so. Therefore, the patient might believe that the most cost-efficient option on his fixed income would be to have surgery despite the fact that he has perfectly acceptable nonsurgical options available.

The insurance company knows it only has to cover his expenses for three more years, so it might save money by paying for the extra medications during that period in order to avoid paying for the entire cost of the penile prosthesis. Once the patient is on Medicare, the company has no more responsibility. Medicare, on the other hand, would like the patient to have a penile prosthesis placed prior to reaching sixty-six. They would then be responsible for no costs unless the device ever failed and had to be replaced. Therefore, you can see that cost calculations are complex.

Regardless of payer, the approximate *total* cost of different options is detailed in the list on page 289.

Note that the cost of some treatments is based on the frequency of usage. This is an advantage of a constriction ring, a vacuum constriction device, or surgery. A VCD is virtually indestructible, especially if a hand pump is used instead of one powered electrically. On the other hand, oral medications and injectables don't cost much for one use, but for men using them on a frequent basis, the costs can soar.

Counseling	$500-$3,000 (depending on frequency and intensity required)
Oral medication	$8-$15 per pill (may be broken into pieces to decrease cost)
Constriction ring	$10-$121
MUSE	$25-$30 per use
Vacuum Constriction Device	$350-$500 (one-time cost)
Intracorporeal injections	$3.50-$35 per injection
Penile prosthesis	$6,000-$15,000 (one-time cost unless revision is required)
Vascular surgery	$8,000-$15,000

ADVANTAGES AND DISADVANTAGES

Defining the best treatment depends on what you mean by best. Oral medications are the best first-line treatment for most men due to their simplicity and the ability to use them only when needed. However, not all men can or will be willing to take oral medications. In an attempt to "cut to the bone," each treatment is summarized in the following paragraphs.

Oral medications are the easiest treatment to begin, requiring only that the physician confirm the patient is an acceptable candidate and write a prescription the patient will have filled. However, they are expensive and carry the risk of a prescription medication.

Counseling is expensive and time-consuming, and it requires substantial emotional effort on the part of the patient and usually his partner. However, counseling can lead to permanent resolution if psychological issues are the primary cause of erectile dysfunction.

Constriction rings and vacuum constriction devices (VCDs) are the safest treatments known to man. In addition, a one-time affordable expenditure enables treatment as frequently as is desired. Unfortunately, they lack spontaneity and provide an erection that appears unnatural to some couples due to either coolness of the penis or the presence of the constriction ring. They are usually only tolerated by stable couples who are willing to put in the effort and who are not bothered by their mechanical nature.

Intracorporeal pharmacotherapy (ICP) is successful for most men who are willing to try it. However, the idea of sticking a needle into the penis is not exactly a great marketing advantage. The MUSE system allows use of the same medication without the needle, but it doesn't work for many patients. The cost of ICP is variable, from as low as $3.50 for generic low-dose **tri-mix** to $35 for the brand-name option **Caverject**. Some couples regard the injections as being non-spontaneous and feel that having to stop to inject the penis can ruin the mood. On the contrary, some couples actually integrate the injection into their foreplay. If men are self-conscious and don't want their partner to know they require help with erections, they can actually excuse themselves into the restroom for an injection. It can be accomplished in the time that they would normally take to empty their bladder. By the time he crawls in bed and romance begins, she probably will notice the erection rise at the time it would have naturally occurred, giving the impression that all is well with the world. Complications such as priapism, fibrosis, or pain are uncommon, but with them comes a little more cause for concern than with the simpler treatments.

Penile prostheses are expensive and require surgery on a sensitive area. However, they are very reliable and have the highest satisfaction of any treatment available. Like any mechanical device, they are not foolproof and can break down (or get infected). In the event of failure, a return to the operating room is the only solution.

Penile **revascularization** and **venous ligation surgery** are helpful only in rare situations. Failure rates and costs are both high. However, for the occasional patient with a surgically correctable problem, they provide the only cure available for erectile dysfunction due to physical causes.

Most importantly, get rid of the cigarettes. They're killing the rest of you, and the penis is just the first casualty.

Finally, don't forget the simpler things. Lifestyle changes are often free, or even better yet, might actually save you money! Giving up smoking will provide the money to cover a romantic evening with your partner. Getting back on that treadmill sitting unused in the corner of the basement may help get things moving in the bedroom as well. As the rest of your body recovers health, the penis will surely follow.

MAKING THE CHOICE

George Harris was a forty-two-year-old insulin-dependent diabetic who responded well to Viagra for three years after developing erectile dysfunction. However, as his diabetes worsened, so did the erectile dysfunction. Even increasing to the maximal dose of 100 milligrams didn't allow satisfactory erections after a while. His primary care physician recommended a urology consultation to consider injections.

George's brother, Fred, was my patient as well. As diabetics, they had both experienced complications from the disease, including erectile dysfunction. Fred was older and the diabetes had been present longer, causing more damage. He had been through the gamut—oral medications, MUSE, a VCD, and injections. He had responded to each treatment for a short period, but none of these options had ever provided a satisfactory erection for him. It had become clear at some point that Fred would not be adequately treated by anything other than a prosthesis, so I referred him to a partner for surgery. Two years after implantation, he used it once a week like clockwork and was pleased with his outcome.

When George arrived in the office, we discussed all the above options. I normally recommend that men try either a VCD or ICP in this situation, but George didn't look favorably on either. He had discussed the possibilities with Fred, who had convinced him that a prosthesis was the only way to go. I couldn't let the younger brother move straight to surgery without being fully informed, however, so he agreed to meet with the impotence coordinator to make sure he fully understood his options. He reviewed each option attentively and respectfully and then reiterated that a penile prosthesis was his choice. Since his decision was fully informed, I made the referral and arranged for placement of a prosthesis. Fred and George both report that the Harris family is doing its part in the battle to keep America sexually active.

Remember that the initial choice made doesn't have to be permanent, unless that choice is surgery. Don't be hesitant to try different options before deciding on what meets your needs the best. However, don't be trapped into believing that you have to try every option prior to having surgery to place a penile implant. The Harris brothers above used both approaches. Fred tried everything before finding that a penile prosthesis was the only satisfactory option for him. His younger brother, George, didn't need to try them all. He knew what he wanted to do. My responsibility was to make sure he was making a fully informed decision. Once that was assured, George was an excellent candidate for prosthesis surgery.

Surgery isn't the "last hope." It is a very acceptable treatment option that, as noted, is known for patient satisfaction greater than that for *any* other form of therapy for erectile dysfunction, including medications. Therefore, if you are not satisfied with the other options, you should explore the possibility of penile prosthesis surgery with a reputable urologist.

A logical description of the progression men might go through in treating erectile dysfunction involves the **progressive treatment model**, which compares management of erectile dysfunction to management of *osteoarthritis*. They point out that oral medications are usually first line treatment of either disease. Anti-inflammatory drugs such as ibuprofen or aspirin are used for arthritis, while erectile dysfunction patients usually try oral medications such as Viagra first. Second- and third-line therapy for arthritis might involve physical therapy, steroid injection into the painful joint, or insertion of a small scope into the joint for minor correction. Likewise, sex therapy, VCDs, MUSE, or injection of vasoactive medications into the nonfunctioning "joint" might be second- or third-line therapy for erectile dysfunction. Finally, prosthetic joint replacement for arthritis that doesn't respond to simpler measures is comparable to prosthesis placement for erectile dysfunction. However, keep in mind that patients who are having severe enough problems with either disorder might simply skip right to surgery if it becomes clear that nonsurgical management is not going to be adequate.

KEY POINTS

- The goal-oriented approach to treatment will meet the needs of most men with erectile dysfunction.
- An open dialogue between patient and physician is crucial to management of erectile dysfunction. The physician's responsibility is to make information, support, and treatment available, but you share in the responsibility. You must communicate your needs to the physician if you hope to have him know how to help you. If you leave him guessing what you are thinking, you will share the blame if the outcome is not to your satisfaction.
- Most patients do not need diagnostic testing in order to successfully manage erectile dysfunction.
- The progressive treatment model demonstrates how treatment of erectile dysfunction is similar to other illnesses, such as arthritis. Erectile dysfunction should be managed with the seriousness of any other illness.
- Once managed, every individual can enjoy a fulfilling and satisfying sex life with his partner.

Conclusion
Keeping Up Hope

We cannot, by an effort of the will, either command or restrain the erection of the penis.

—Robert Whytt, *An Essay on the Vital and Other Involuntary Motions of Animals*

*I*t has been my goal to cover the issues involved in preventing and treating erectile dysfunction as clearly as possible. After reading these pages, I hope you are reassured that your sex life can be healthy and active for as long as you wish. There is no reason to accept erectile dysfunction as long as you are healthy enough to enjoy sex.

Now it is time for you to take charge of your sexual health. If you are starting to see signs of trouble, it is time to look at your overall health. Get back in shape, stop smoking if you haven't already done so, and make sure your mental health is not ignored. It is every bit as important as your physical health.

If the simple treatments don't work, don't be shy about asking your physician about a trial of oral medications. Look into counseling or other mental health therapy if there are issues that need to be addressed. If there is still no improvement, don't give up. Injections, MUSE, VCDs, and surgery offer hope where previously there was none. To summarize, do whatever it takes to achieve success. As you now know, the limitations can be overcome if you make up your mind to do so.

The future is bright for men with erectile dysfunction with the options available today, and research continues to offer new options. Whereas current management of erectile dysfunction involves overcoming the symptom to achieve an erection when needed, the future might offer a true cure. If that goal is realized, men previously reliant on treatment might be able to return to full sexual function and have erections available on demand.

NEUROMUSCULAR RESEARCH

The third thousandth year of the Christian era will bring at least a
clarification, if not a solution, of many problems of sex and love.
—Theodore Reik, *Psychology of Sex Relations*, 1945

Researchers around the globe continue to seek better treatments for erectile dysfunction. Their efforts are focused on every possible target and someday may involve future approaches we can't even imagine today. Pharmaceutical companies continue to seek better medications. The most important current goal is to hasten onset of action so that a man could take a pill on the way to the bedroom and his erection would be ready as he goes through the threshold.

However, although the current medications are amazingly effective, some men still aren't adequately treated by a pill. Although side effects are uncommon, they will never be eliminated for any drug. However, further decreasing side effects and eliminating drug interactions like those involving phosphodiesterase (PDE) inhibitors and nitrates will allow more men to be treated with oral medications.

The medications currently available in America work on a part of the erection mechanism that a generation ago we didn't even know existed. Who knows what other chemical actions play a role that has not been identified yet? We may find new enzymes that could be targeted by new drugs. In the future, we may target the brain or other parts of the erection mechanism that have heretofore been thought inaccessible.

Nerve regeneration research is currently under way for many neurological conditions. This approach may lead to a better understanding of recovery of nerve function to the penis. Men who have had nerve damage from trauma, surgery, diabetes, or neurological diseases stand to benefit the most if this avenue shows promise in treating erectile dysfunction.

Some surgeons are using the *sural nerve*, a relatively unimportant nerve harvested from the leg, to graft the severed ends of the penile nerves together during a radical retropubic prostatectomy. Their early results indicate that this may allow the nerves to regenerate and erections to return. We may also find that gels or sutures might accomplish the same thing without the major reconstruction required for sural nerve grafts. In addition, muscles, vein grafts, or animal grafts such as *small intestine submucosa* might also be able to achieve this. *Stem cell research* (which has been so politically divisive) may someday also play a role in nerve regeneration to the penis.

Scientists in many different disciplines are actively pursuing research on nerve regeneration in order to treat diseases as varied as multiple sclerosis and spinal cord injury. Their efforts will inevitably affect the way urologists treat erectile dysfunction at some point. Promising examples include *Neurotropins*, chemicals that have recently been identified that stimulate nerve regeneration. Another, *nerve growth factor*, may be one way to help those with diabetic neuropathy (nerve damage).

Many researchers use phosphodiesterase inhibitors, prostaglandin injections, MUSE, or VCDs to hasten recovery of erections following prostatectomy. According to my friend and colleague, Dr. Craig Zippe, these interventions provide blood flow needed to maintain health of the corporal tissue and may stimulate unknown chemical factors in the corpora cavernosae.[1]

RESTORING BLOOD FLOW

> He who ceases to be better ceases to be good.
> —generally attributed to Oliver Cromwell

Venous insufficiency is the cause of more erectile dysfunction than is commonly believed. Prevention will be the mainstay of its management. For example, it appears that losing connection of the nerves to the cavernous smooth muscle through surgery, trauma, or diabetes, causes this muscle to *atrophy*, or shrink. This is the same concept that happens to a muscle anywhere whose nerve is severed. This shrinkage contributes to venous insufficiency and makes treatment more difficult, as the condition worsens over time. Finding a way to stimulate these muscles artificially could theoretically prevent this damage from occurring. The work of Dr. Zippe and others mentioned above seeks to meet that goal.

Pharmacologically induced *angiogenesis* (growth of new blood supply) could restore normal blood flow in the future. *Vascular endothelial growth factor (VEGF)* or similar growth factors could be used to cause regrowth of penile veins or arteries. In addition, as newer treatments for arteriosclerosis are improved, penile blood flow will gain from the overall improvement in vascular status. If that occurs, the penis could serve as a barometer of recovery in much the same way that it now serves as a barometer of overall health and deterioration.

Finally, gene therapy offers promise for several parts of the puzzle, but it is likely to be most beneficial for men with abnormalities of the erectile tissue. Gene therapy has the potential to play a particularly significant role in venous insufficiency if the theory is correct that abnormal sinusoids can be repaired using this method. One can only imagine the promise this holds of restoring erectile tissues.

HORMONAL RESEARCH

Since hormones appear to be more important in female sexual response, most research progress will probably be made for women in the foreseeable future. Particularly appealing would be the development of an androgen (male-type hormone) that doesn't cause the side effects of today's testosterone preparations. The most significant side effect currently is *masculinization*, which for women has greatly limited the role of testosterone replacement therapy. Women wishing to be more sexually active don't find treatment appealing if the treatment causes them to look like a man.

In addition, it is likely that there are hormones involved in the sexual response of both genders that haven't even been identified. Targeting these might yield unforeseen benefits.

PREVENTION

The real hope for the future may lie in prevention. It is naive to think that we could wipe out all disease and pestilence; yet progress continues for many of the diseases that contribute to erectile dysfunction. We can now control hypertension (high blood pressure), diabetes, mental disorders, high cholesterol, and many other chronic disease states that cause impotence. Newer medications for many diseases cause fewer side effects than their predecessors. Smoking may eventually become extinct.

Treatments for prostate and colon cancer result in far fewer cases of impotence now than even a decade ago. As these treatments are refined, potency is one of the most significant parameters used to judge improvement. There is even more room for improvement in female pelvic surgery as preservation of sexual function is prioritized.

Finally, as our understanding of vitamins and supplements improves, we hope to find scientifically sound, safe, natural products that will help preserve sexual function. Since most people would prefer a natural, effective, and safe product to a man-made treatment, success with the product is guaranteed if ever such a substance is identified.

A FINAL WORD

O most lame and impotent conclusion!
—Shakespeare, *Othello*, act 2, scene 3

We know a lot, but there is still too much we don't know about sexual function. The most important thing we know is that it is as crucial to human health as any other function. Fortunately, with the advances made during our lifetimes there are very few men whose erectile dysfunction can't be treated. Twenty years ago, the same could not be said.

Whether you choose to be sexually active or not, know that the choice is yours and your partner's alone. If you need treatment in order to act on that choice, you have several excellent options readily available. May your choices bring you and your mate a lifetime of intimacy that meets both your needs and fulfills your dreams.

Notes

PREFACE

1. D. R. Smith, ed., *General Urology*, 5th ed. (Los Altos, Calif.: Lange Medical Publications, 1966).

INTRODUCTION

1. H. A. Feldman et al., "Impotence and Its Medical and Psychological Correlates: Results of the *Massachusetts Male Aging Study*," *Journal of Urology* 151 (1994): 54.
2. Ibid.
3. Alfred Kinsey, *Sexual Behavior in the Human Male* (Philadelphia: W. B. Saunders, 1948).

CHAPTER 1

1. Gen. 20:2–18.
2. 1 Kings 1:1–30.
3. Meredith Campbell and Hartwell Harrison, *Campbell's Urology* (Philadelphia: W. B. Saunders, 1970).

CHAPTER 3

1. Leslie Schover and Anthony J. Thomas, *Overcoming Infertility* (New York: J. Wiley, 2000).

2. P. Mathur, K. Prabhu, and H. L. Khamesra, "Polyorchidism Revisited," *Pediatric Surgery International* 14 (2002): 449–50.

3. J. K. Chon, "The Cost Value of Medical versus Surgical Hormonal Therapy for Metastatic Prostate Cancer," *Journal of Urology* 164 (2000): 735–37.

4. Robert E. Reiter and Jean de Kernion, *Campbell's Urology*, 8th ed. (Philadelphia: W. B. Saunders, 2002), p. 3010.

5. Elizabeth Miller et al., "Tomato Products, Lycopene, and Prostate Cancer Risk," *Urologic Clinics of North America* 29 (2002): 83–93.

CHAPTER 4

1. Quoted in Larry Katzenstein, *Viagra* (New York: CMD Publishing, 2001).

CHAPTER 5

1. Richard Milstein and Julian Slowinski, *The Sexual Male: Problems and Solutions* (New York: W. W. Norton, 1999), pp. 211–15.

2. Ibid.

3. Davey Smith, S. Frankel, and J. Yarnell, "Sex and Death: Are They Related? Findings from the Caerphilly Cohort Study," *British Medical Journal* 315 (1997): 1641–44.

4. Quoted in William Gee, "A History of Surgical Treatment of Impotence," *Urology* 5 (1975): 3.

5. Milstein and Slowinski, *The Sexual Male*, pp. 73–87.

6. Ibid.

7. A. D. Seftel and S. E. Althof, "Rapid Ejaculation," *Current Urologic Opinions* 1 (2000): 302–306.

8. Dave Barry, *Dave Barry's Complete Guide to Guys* (New York: Random House, 1995).

9. Statistics from J. Stephen Jones. *Urology Secrets* (Philadelphia: Hanley and Belfus, 2002).

CHAPTER 6

1. American Cancer Society, *Facts and Figures* (2003).

2. Derek Lipman, *Snoring from A to ZZZZ: Proven Cures for the Night's Worst Nuisance* (Portland: Spencer Press, 1996).
3. Patrick Walsh, *Dr. Patrick Walsh's Guide to Surviving Prostate Cancer* (New York: Warner Books, 2001).
4. Meredith Campbell and Hartwell Harrison, *Campbell's Urology* (Philadelphia: W. B. Saunders, 1970).
5. Joseph Cohen, *The Penis Book* (Cologne: Koneemann Verlagsgesellschaft, 1999).

CHAPTER 7

1. P. H. Brenot, *Male Impotence—A Historical Perspective* (L'Esprit du Temps, 1994).
2. Roy Porter, *The Greatest Benefit to Mankind: A Medical History of Humanity* (New York: W. W. Norton, 1997), pp. 703–704.

CHAPTER 8

1. William H. Masters and Virginia Johnson, *Human Sexual Response* (Boston: Little, Brown, 1966).
2. E. Laumann, A. Pike, and R. C. Rosen, "The Epidemiology of Erectile Dysfunction: Results from the National Health and Social Life Survey," *International Journal of Impotence Research* 11, suppl. 1 (1999): S60–64.
2. J. R. Berman, "Female Sexual Dysfunction," *Urologic Clinics of North America* (2001): 405–16.

CHAPTER 10

1. William H. Masters and Virginia Johnson, *Human Sexual Response* (Boston: Little, Brown, 1966).

CHAPTER 11

1. William R. Fair and Willet Whitmore Jr., "Lecture: Back to the Future—The Role of Complementary Medicine in Urology," *Journal of Urology* 162 (1999): 411.
2. G. S. Gerber, "Saw Palmetto for the Treatment of Men with Lower Urinary Tract Symptoms," *Journal of Urology* 163 (2000): 1408–12.
3. A. H. Fiefer, N. E. Fleshner, and L. Klotz, "Analytical Accuracy and Reli-

ability of Commonly Used Nutritional Supplements in Prostate Disease," *Journal of Urology* 168 (2002): 150–54.

4. E. J. Small, M. W. Froelich, and R. Bok, *Journal of Clinical Oncology* 18 (2000): 3595–3603.

5. Mark Moyad, "Dietary Supplements and Other Complementary Medicines for Erectile Dysfunction: What Do I Tell My Patients?" *Urologic Clinics of North America* 29, no. 1 (2002): 11–22.

6. Ambrose Bierce, *The Devil's Dictionary* (1906; reprint, New York: Dover Publications, 1993), p. 51.

CHAPTER 12

1. Larry Katzenstein, *Viagra: The Remarkable Story of the Discovery and Launch* (Taiwan: Medical Information Press, 2001).

CHAPTER 13

1. Gregory Broderick and Tom Lue. *Campbell's Urology*, 8th ed. (Philadelphia: W. B. Saunders, 2002), pp. 1655–56.

CHAPTER 14

1. Drogo K. Montague and Kenneth Angermeier, "Penile Prosthesis Implantation," *Urologic Clinics of North America* 28 (2001): 355–61.
2. Ibid.
3. Ibid.
4. Ibid.
5. Ibid.

CHAPTER 15

1. Gregory Broderick and Tom Lue, *Campbell's Urology*, 8th ed. (Philadelphia: W. B. Saunders, 2002), pp. 1690–95.

CONCLUSION

1. Craig D. Zippe, Personal communication, February 24, 2003.

Appendix A
Resources

$\mathcal{T}$he best source of information regarding erectile dysfunction, as well as smoking cessation and the other health issues covered in this book, is your primary care physician. A local urologist or sex therapist can also help specifically with sexual health issues. However, the following is a list of resources you may find helpful as well.

American Association for Marriage and Family Therapy
112 South Alfred Street
Alexandria, VA 22314-3061
Phone: (703) 838-9808
Fax: (703) 838-9805

American Association of Sex Educators, Counselors, and Therapists
P.O. Box 5488
Richmond, VA 23220-0488
E-mail: aasect@aasect.org

Sexual Function Health Council
American Foundation for Urologic Disease
1128 North Charles Street
Baltimore, MD 21201

**The Sexuality Information and Education Council
of the United States (SIECUS)**
130 West 42nd Street, Suite 350
New York, NY 10036
Phone: (212) 819-9770

Society for the Scientific Study of Sexuality
P.O. Box 416
Allentown, PA 18105-0416 U.S.A.
Phone: (610) 530-2483
Fax: (610) 530-2485
E-mail: thesociety@inetmail.att.net

Appendix B
Definition of Terms

ACTIS RING. Brand of constriction ring that is softer and less likely to pull hair than most versions.

ALPROSTADIL. One of several vasodilating agents available to treat erectile dysfunction when injected into the penile shaft.

ANEJACULATION. An absence of semen at ejaculation.

ANORGASMIA. Complete absence of climax or orgasm.

APOMORPHINE. Generic name for a drug that is available for erectile dysfunction in many countries as the brand name Uprima or Ixense. Acts at the brain level, affecting an aspect of the erection cascade different from those affect by phosphodiesterase (PDE) inhibitors.

ARTERIOGRAPHY. Injection of dye into the penile arteries, used to confirm injury or obstruction.

ARTERIOSCLEROSIS. Hardening of the arteries, leading to inadequate blood flow. When arteriosclerosis occurs in the blood vessels supplying vital organs such as the brain or heart, life-threatening problems can occur. Arteriosclerosis also affects the penile arteries, resulting in erectile dysfunction.

AUTO-INFLATION. A spontaneous erection of the cylinders of a penile prosthesis based purely on excess pressure exerted on the reservoir.

"BI-MIX" OR "TRI-MIX." Various combinations of vasodilators used for intracorporeal pharmacotherapy.

BIOPSY. See **Prostate biopsy**.

BULBOCAVERNOSUS REFLEX. A test performed with an examining finger inside the anal sphincter, which should contract if neurological reflexes are intact. If absent, a neurological deficit is suspected of playing a role in erectile dysfunction.

CAVERJECT. One of the brand name versions of alprostadil, used for intracorporeal pharmacotherapy.

CAVERNOSOGRAPHY. Radiographic imaging of the corpora cavernosae; performed in order to demonstrate enlarged veins exiting the penis in patients suspected of venous insufficiency.

CLITORIS. The female version of a penis. The most significant organ for sexual stimulation in most women.

CONSTRICTION RING. Soft latex ring designed to operate like a tourniquet. When tightened around the base of the penis, it helps maintain enough blood inside the corporal bodies to maintain an erection. Especially useful for men using a vacuum constriction device or for men with venous insufficiency.

CORPUS CAVERNOSUM (plural CORPORA CAVERNOSAE or CORPORAL BODIES). The two cylinders that extend the length of the penis, from their connection deep in the bony pelvis to the tip. Filling of these cylinders creates the rigidity required for an erection.

CORPUS SPONGIOSUM. The third cylinder of the penis, located on the undersurface. Holds the urethra and spreads out at the end of the penis in order to cover the corporal bodies. This expansion is called the glans penis.

CYCLIC GMP. An enzyme related to the development of an erection. When the enzyme phosphodiesterase type 5 is blocked, this enzyme accumulates and continues to allow the erection to persist.

CYSTOSCOPY. Placement of a small scope through the urethra into the urinary bladder. The scope is a relatively soft, flexible tube with fiber optic fibers running through it that allows the urologist to see the inside of the urethra, prostate, and urinary bladder.

DETUMESCENCE. Deflation of an erection due to the exit of blood from the penis, resulting in internal pressure inadequate to maintain further rigidity.

DIABETES MELLITUS, A condition that results in elevated levels of sugar (glucose) in the bloodstream. Related to many complications, including erectile dysfunction.

DOPPLER ULTRASOUND. Radiologic test that assesses penile blood flow.

DYSPAREUNIA. Painful intercourse.

EDEX. One of the brand name versions of alprostadil; used for intracorporeal pharmacotherapy.

EJACULATE. A word used as a verb to denote the release of semen from the penis, or as a noun to describe that fluid. The event is called ejaculation.

EJACULATION. Word originally meaning "to throw a dart." Therefore an ejaculation is the physical expulsion of semen from the urethra.

EMISSION. Release of semen into the urethra that initiates ejaculation.

EPIDIDYMIS. A small sack on the back of the testis where sperm cells mature prior to their release to the seminal vesicles.

ERECTILE DYSFUNCTION (ED). The inability to achieve or maintain an erection.

FIBROSIS. A term for scarring. Penile fibrosis can inhibit erections or make them curved.

FORSKOLIN. A natural vasodilator recently introduced for intracorporeal pharmacotherapy.

GLANS PENIS. The expansion of the corpus spongiosum that spreads over the corporal bodies as the "head" of the penis. Holds the nerve fibers that give the penis its sensitivity.

GOAL-ORIENTED APPROACH. Treatment of erectile dysfunction based on meeting the patient's needs rather than on obtaining a specific causative diagnosis. Treatment options are usually the same, so treatment is offered irrespective of the underlying cause in most instances.

HYPOGONADISM. Condition in which production of testosterone is low ("hypo").

IIEF (INTERNATIONAL INDEX OF ERECTILE FUNCTION). The standard sexual questionnaire required for most medical publications reporting research involving erectile dysfunction. It is also used to quantify the degree of erectile difficulty. The IIEF started out as a fifteen-question list, but its little brother, the IIEF-5, cuts right to the bone with five questions (listed in chapter 7, "Sex Scores: Questionnaires").

INTRACORPOREAL PHARMACOTHERAPY (ICP). Injection of medications into the penile shaft in order to create blood flow, and thereby an erection.

IMPOTENCE. See **erectile dysfunction**.

IMPOTENCE COORDINATOR. Ancillary health care provider trained in impotence education. Can be extremely useful in all phases of care, helping patients assess treatment options.

LEYDIG CELLS. Little cellular testosterone factories inside the testis.

LIBIDO. Desire for sexual activity.

MALLEABLE (SEMIRIGID) PROSTHESES. Noninflatable penile prostheses with few or no moving parts also called *rod prostheses.*

MUSE (MEDICATED URETHRAL SYSTEM FOR ERECTION). A plastic applicator the size of a matchstick that is inserted about an inch into the urethra and squeezed to deliver a small (1 × 3-millimeter) semisolid alprostadil pellet.

NEW PARTNER SYNDROME. Erectile dysfunction in a man involved with a new partner that relates to performance anxiety.

NOCTURNAL PENILE TUMESCENCE (NPT). The assessment of penile erections during sleep. The presence of erections indicates that the patient is capable of achieving an erection at least in certain circumstances but doesn't necessarily mean the problem is psychological.

NITRATES. Vasodilators used to treat heart problems that interact with phosphodiesterase inhibitors in a manner that can be fatal. In combination they actually augment each other's effects on blood vessels, leading to a dangerous dilation of blood vessels, thereby decreasing blood pressure to dangerous levels. In addition, these changes are not easily reversible, so the drop in blood pressure can be life-threatening; in short, the combination can kill.

NITRIC OXIDE (NO). a neurotransmitter (chemical that is used by a nerve to cause its action) that releases cyclic GMP, which allows the sinusoids to fill under pressure.

OBSTRUCTIVE SLEEP APNEA (OSA). A condition resulting from a narrowed airway intake during sleep. An early sign is snoring, but severe cases involve intermittent episodes when the body may become starved for oxygen.

ORGASM. The neurological event experienced as the pleasurable climax to sexual activity. This sensation is independent of emission or ejaculation.

PAPAVERINE. One of the agents used for vasodilation during intracorporeal pharmacotherapy.

PELVIC STEAL SYNDROME. Shunting of blood flow from the penis to the pelvic muscles, causing early detumescence.

PENILE PROSTHESES. Devices implanted inside the penis that stiffen it mechanically instead of through physiological processes. Although surgery is required, patient satisfaction is greater for those who receive penile prostheses than for any other form of impotence therapy.

PERFORMANCE ANXIETY. Anxiety or stress due to a fear of failure or unworthiness. This fear of failure often accompanies erectile dysfunction and may be the final issue to cause men to be unable to perform.

PEYRONIE'S DISEASE. A disorder caused by fibrosis (scarring) of the tunica albuginea, which can cause penile curvature, pain, or erectile dysfunction.

PHENTOLAMINE. One of the agents used for vasodilation during intracorporeal pharmacotherapy.

PRIAPISM. A painful, prolonged erection that causes permanent damage to the erectile tissues if allowed to persist beyond a few hours.

PHOSPHODIESTERASE (PDE) INHIBITORS. Chemicals that prevent the degradation of cyclic GMP and allow the penile arteries to remain open and an erection to be maintained more readily. Viagra, Cialis, and Vardenafil are the options either available or under review at the time of writing.

PLACEBO EFFECT. The principle that causes people to respond to treatment based on the knowledge that they are supposed to improve simply because they have been treated. This explains why some people get better when receiving a placebo (fake) treatment.

PROGRESSIVE TREATMENT MODEL. An idea that compares management of erectile dysfunction to management of osteoarthritis. Oral medications are usually the first-line treatment for either disease. Second- and third-line therapy for arthritis might involve physical therapy, steroid injection into the painful joint, or insertion of a small scope into the joint for minor correction. Likewise, sex therapy, vacuum constriction devices, MUSE, or intracorporeal pharmacotherapy might be second- or third-line therapy for erectile dysfunction. Finally, prosthetic joint replacement for arthritis that doesn't respond to simpler measures is comparable to prosthesis placement for erectile dysfunction.

PROSTAGLANDIN E1. Another term for alprostadil, one of the vasodilators used for penile injection and also used in MUSE.

PROSTATE. The gland in a man's pelvis (beneath the bladder) that produces much of the semen but plays no known direct role in erections.

PUDENDAL ARTERIES AND VEINS. Vessels that supply blood to the penis (arteries) and carry it back out (veins).

PROSTATE BIOPSY. An office-based procedure used to obtain small samples (biopsies) of prostate tissue through a needle under local anesthesia.

PSA (PROSTATE SPECIFIC ANTIGEN). A blood test that is used in combination with a rectal examination in order to optimize the early detection of prostate cancer.

PROSTATITIS. An inflammatory condition of the prostate that may be due to infection but is more commonly due simply to irritation—sort of an arthritis of the prostate.

RADICAL PROSTATECTOMY. Operation that removes a cancerous prostate. Due to the presence of the penile nerves immediately adjacent to the prostate, erectile dysfunction can occur due to injury during this operation.

RAPID (PREMATURE) EJACULATION. Achieving ejaculation or orgasm more rapidly than desired. There is no absolute time value that accurately defines rapid ejaculation, so it is based on individual interpretation.

REFRACTORY PERIOD. The time following orgasm when men are unable to achieve erection or repeat orgasm. This time normally becomes progressively longer as men age.

RETROGRADE EJACULATION. Release of semen backward (retrograde) into the bladder instead of out the urethra.

REVASCULARIZATION. Operation that bypasses obstruction of arteries, allowing normal blood flow to be reestablished to the penis.

RIGISCAN. A device that assesses nocturnal penile tumescence in the home.

SCROTUM. The sac that contains the spermatic cords and the testes.

SEMEN. The fluid released during male orgasm or ejaculation. Sperm cells actually compose less than 1 percent of seminal volume. The remainder is fluid produced in the prostate, the seminal vesicles, and other secondary sex organs.

SEMINAL VESICLES. Sacs that sit behind the bladder, attached to the prostate. Over half of the ejaculate is produced by these hidden secondary sex glands.

SEMINIFEROUS TUBULES. Hundreds of coils inside the testis that can stretch out to about a yard long. Sperm cells are born in the tubules.

SEXUAL RESPONSE CYCLE. The stages of sexual behavior described by Masters and Johnson: *excitement, plateau, orgasm*, and *resolution*. Sexual activity will not always involve a progression through all four stages, especially for women. Sildenafil (Viagra). The first PDE-5 inhibitor approved for the treatment of erectile dysfunction.

SINUSOIDS. Sacs inside the corporal bodies that fill with blood, making the penis inflated and rigid.

SNAP GAUGE. A device wrapped around the penis during sleep, held in place with a Velcro fastener. Different layers of the device rupture as a result of different erection forces during the night, leaving a trail of evidence regarding rigidity during asleep.

SPANISH FLY. A reputed aphrodisiac made from the ground wings of the insect otherwise known as the blister beetle. There is no scientific evidence it works, but there is plenty of proof it causes abdominal pain, seizures, rectal bleeding, erosion of mucosal surfaces (the lining of the organs), and internal bleeding. Death can occur from these side effects.

SPECTATORING. A situation often experienced in men with severe performance anxiety, where the man describes the sensation of watching himself developing a fear of failure.

SPERMATIC CORDS. Woven ropes of arteries, veins, muscles, nerves, and other tissues that connect the testes to the rest of the body. The most important and strongest structure in the spermatic cord is the vas deferens.

SQUEEZE TECHNIQUE. Attempting to interrupt orgasm by firmly squeezing the glans penis when a sense of inevitability approaches. This takes advantage of the nervous system's tendency to shut down sensation when overwhelmed.

STAMP TEST (POSTAGE STAMP TEST). A simple method to assess whether an erection occurs during sleep. A roll of stamps is secured to itself around the base of the penis. A rupture at the perforations indicates that an erection occurred during sleep.

TADALAFIL (CIALIS). A PDE-5 inhibitor that has a significantly longer duration of action than the other PDE-5 inhibitors, lasting two to three days; therefore regarded as the "weekend drug."

TESTOSTERONE. Male hormone produced primarily in the testes. Its role in erections is not completely understood, but appears to involve mainly libido.

TITRATE. Adjusting a medication dosage to determine the proper amount.

TUMESCENCE. Another term meaning "erection."

TUNICA ALBUGINEA. The tough, outer fascial layer that surrounds each corpus cavernosum. It provides the strength to allow an erection instead of simply stretching when the corporal bodies fill under pressure.

TURP (TRANSURETHRAL RESECTION OF THE PROSTATE). Operation for prostate enlargement to create a larger opening through the prostate to allow easier urination.

UPRIMA. See **apomorphine**.

URETHRA. The tube that carries urine and semen through the corpus spongiosum out the tip of the penis.

VACUUM CONSTRICTION DEVICE (VCD). A cylinder designed to create a vacuum around the penis. Negative pressure inside the cylinder causes blood to flow into the corpora cavernosae. When the penis becomes full enough to become erect, a band is allowed to gently constrict around the base of the penis so the pressure remains long enough for intercourse.

VAGINA. The female primary sex organ.

VAGINISMUS. Uncontrolled contractions of the pelvic and vaginal muscles than can cause dyspareunia.

VARDENAFIL (LEVITRA). A phosphodiesterase inhibitor with little effect on PDE-6, thus lacking the minor visual side effects associated with other PDE-5 inhibitors.

VAS DEFERENS. The thick tube that carries sperm on the first part of its journey from the epididymis.

VASECTOMY. A minor operation to remove a small segment of the vas deferens in order to block the exit of sperm cells, rendering a man incapable of procreation; performed through one or two small incisions in the scrotum using local anesthesia. Minimally invasive options include the no-scalpel or percutaneous methods.

VASOCONSTRICTION. The opposite of vasodilation. A medication or other agent that causes blood vessels to narrow is a vasoconstrictor.

VASODILATION. The opening of a blood vessel to allow filling of an organ. This is central to producing an erection.

VENOUS INSUFFICIENCY. Abnormality of the veins exiting the penis that allows blood to flow out too easily, preventing the pressure inside the corporal bodies from reaching or maintaining adequate levels for erection.

VENOUS LIGATION SURGERY. An operation to tie off veins that allow blood to escape the penis too readily.

VICIOUS CYCLE. A situation in which one problem perpetuates another, while the second starts the process over again.

VULVA. The external genitalia of the female.

YOHIMBINE. The product of a tree bark that has been used to treat erectile dysfunction for decades. Evidence of its effectiveness is weak.

Index